THE FRENCH BEAUTY SOLUTION

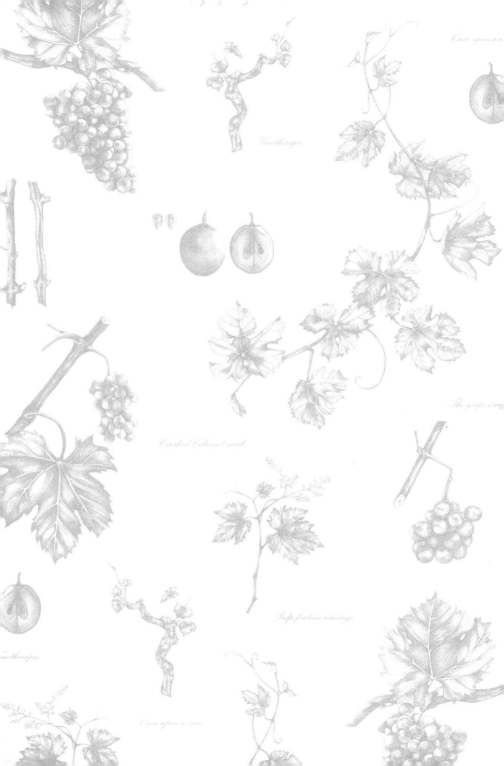

THE
French Beauty
SOLUTION

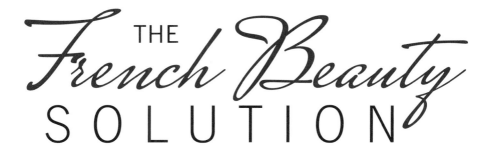

TIME-TESTED SECRETS TO LOOK AND
FEEL BEAUTIFUL INSIDE AND OUT

MATHILDE THOMAS

AVERY

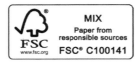

An imprint of Penguin Random House LLC
375 Hudson Street
New York, New York 10014

LIBRARY OF CONGRESS CATALOGING-IN-PUBLICATION DATA
Cathiard-Thomas, Mathilde.
The French beauty solution : time-tested secrets to look and feel beautiful inside and out / Mathilde Thomas.
pages cm
ISBN 978-1-592-40951-8 (hardback)
1. Skin—Care and hygiene. 2. Women—Health and hygiene.
3. Beauty, Personal. 4. Self-care, Health. I. Title.
RL87.C38 2015
646.7'2—dc23
2015003934

Printed in the United States of America

5   7   9   10   8   6

BOOK DESIGN BY SPRING HOTELING

Penguin
Random
House

TO BERTRAND.

TO PAUL, LOUISE, AND MARION.

CONTENTS

CONTENTS

INTRODUCTION

I grew up in Grenoble, a French village nestled at the foot of the French Alps where the air was pure and clean and the mountain water icy crisp. My parents, Daniel and Florence Cathiard, my younger sister, Alice, and I lived on a farm with my maternal grandparents, Yvonne and Maurice, where we tended a vegetable garden and raised chickens and bees. My grandfather took me hiking all over the mountains, pointing out which plants were edible and which mushrooms were toxic, which herbs could cure a tummy ache and which would staunch a wound, which smelled intoxicatingly minty and which were so pungent they made my nose run.

I was lucky to have grown up in that magical place. Even though my grandparents were teachers and spent much of their time correcting papers and reading, they understood how to be one with nature, and they infused my childhood with their knowledge of plants and all growing things.

This was also the place where I learned my first beauty secrets. Even though we lived far from the high-end commercial fashion world of Paris, we had access to dozens of the best beauty regimens right in our own backyard. My grandmother would make a luscious facial mask from the honey in the beehive at the corner of our garden and would always be certain to gently pat some on my cheeks whenever she applied it to her own, because she knew how soothing and clarifying it was. She'd whip up a super-moisturizing and nourishing hair mask from fresh, green, pungent olive oil and rum and we'd sit together, giggling at the scent, till our hair was saturated. She recognized early on how much I loved different fragrances—we would do blind tastings of different herbs, like tarragon, thyme, basil, sage, and mint, and I could always differentiate them, even as a very small child—and wasn't surprised at all when I told her I wanted to work in the beauty business.

As I grew older my grandmother and mother started teaching me their time-tested secrets to looking and feeling beautiful, inside and out—secrets they had learned from their own mothers. I was taught that beauty is not something you turn to in a panic when a wrinkle or pimple appears, but that it's far more important to see it as a ritual, figuring out what routine works best and carrying that with us through our lives. I used those lessons as well as my love for the natural world when my husband, Bertrand, and I founded our skincare company, Caudalie, in 1995, and they were reinforced whenever I returned to the Alps, or went to the vineyard in Bordeaux that my parents bought in 1990.

But it wasn't until Bertrand and I moved with our children from Paris to New York City to grow Caudalie USA in 2010 that I realized that the French attitude toward beauty was not the same as the American one. Learning about and understanding these nuances was absolutely fascinating to me, and as I traveled all over the country, visiting many of the 350-plus Sephora, Nordstrom, and Blue Mercury stores that carry Caudalie products, meeting personally with thousands of customers that year alone, I realized that American women could benefit from a little of my French beauty wisdom. That while millions of them consider beauty a priority in their daily routine, many of their habits are either too complicated, too expensive, too painful, or simply not effective. That is what inspired me to write *The French Beauty Solution*.

Whether I was in Cleveland, Ohio, or Cleveland, Florida, the same issues came up time and again as the women I met candidly discussed their beauty needs and desires. Even though I was asking them specifically about what they wanted from a skincare product, without fail, the conversations always veered away from skincare alone. All my customers wanted the same things: To have wonderful skin, simply and quickly. To age with grace. To lead a healthy lifestyle. To be fit and trim. To know which diets work and which don't. To know how to do a cleanse if they feel the need. To manage their stress. To have a flawlessly made-up face and a doable hairstyle. And to have the kind of effortless beauty and sense of *savoir faire* that seem to be part of a Frenchwoman's DNA.

"How *do* you do it?" these lovely women would ask. "How can I be more, you know, like the French?" I'd laugh and say it really wasn't all that complicated, only to be met with skeptical smiles.

The women I spoke with would tell me how in awe they were of French stylishness, and I'd tell them how much we envied their beautiful teeth and gorgeous hair.

The more I talked to consumers, the more easily I could clarify what precisely differentiated the French beauty philosophies and habits from the American ones. I learned, of course, that one was not necessarily better than the other, but they were indeed *different,* and those differences, I believed, were causing the dissatisfaction among the Americans I spoke to. For the French, our beauty routine is predicated on prevention and upkeep and is regarded as an essential, ongoing investment. What I saw here, however, was much more of a tendency toward the quick solution. I was astonished at the inventiveness of ads extolling the next miracle in a jar—which, because these miracles are nonexistent, often lead women to spend a lot of money on a product only to give up on it when it doesn't solve their problem immediately. And this is precisely what causes so many of the skincare issues women come to talk to me about in the first place—because even the best products need time to work!

Many of these women confessed that they made their beauty choices based on the erroneous notion of no pain/no gain, a deeply American concept that sometimes seems to be conquering the world. They'd tell me about shoes that pinch, crash diets that left them light-headed, and skincare products that irritate their skin—because they felt they had to suffer to be beautiful!

Mon Dieu! I say to that, because the French notion of beauty is quite the opposite. We believe beauty is something to give you *pleasure*. Because when you feel good, you always look good. And what could be more pleasurable than a sinfully rich homemade honey face mask that costs pennies and takes one minute to whip up before leaving your skin shining, smelling delicious, and feeling like velvet? Or how about a glass of delicious red wine with your dinner to help you relax and fill your body with antioxidants that keep aging at bay? The notion of beauty should be, well, *beautiful* and pleasing to you above all. This is the biggest difference between the American and French approaches to beauty solutions.

I've spent the past two decades engrossed in the study of beauty and wellness, continually studying and testing (I've tested some products more than two hundred times!), educating myself on which ingredients pack the most punch while being affordable and as natural and safe as possible—a testament to the lessons I learned growing up.

Even with my upbringing and early lessons in beauty, I would not be writing this book if it weren't for an unexpected encounter I had on a lovely cloudless October day in 1993. My then boyfriend, Bertrand, and I were staying with my parents at their vineyard, Château Smith Haut Lafitte, to help them with the harvest when a group of scientists from the University of Bordeaux paid us a visit—the vineyard is only a fifteen-minute drive from the center of Bordeaux and is a lovely place to visit, especially in the fall. These scientists were studying the chemical molecules and properties of grapes and grapevines, so it made sense for them to come to the place where some of the best grapes in the world are grown in order to make the best wines.

I was twenty-two and very curious to find out what aspects of the grapes had piqued the interest of university researchers, and my father connected the dots for me—he knew that one of the scientists, Professor Joseph Vercauteren, was researching grapes and the vines leftover after the harvest (and he also knew, of course, of my interest in the beauty business and that Bertrand wanted to create his own company). Bertrand and I met them among the grapes, and one of the scientists picked up a few of the grape stalks and a handful of grapes that had fallen on the ground and smiled.

"Do you know that you are throwing away treasures?" he said, meaning the grape seeds that are sent to the distillery after the harvest, once the grapes are pressed.

That was my introduction to Professor Vercauteren, the head of the Pharmacognosy (the study of medicine derived from plants) Laboratory at Bordeaux University of Pharmacy. Nor did I know he was one of the world's leading experts on polyphenols, an antiaging compound found in grapes and grapevines. (I didn't even know what a polyphenol was!) Or that this simple concept would lead to my life's calling: an all-natural beauty revolution based on the luscious, gorgeously ripe purple fruit hanging from the twisting vines that surrounded us.

Professor Vercauteren told Bertrand and me that he had recently discovered that grape polyphenols were the most potent natural antioxidants produced by nature, especially resveratrol, the polyphenol found in grape skins, seeds, and stalks. He believed resveratrol could enhance the life span of cells and help people live longer, healthier lives, which is why he was visiting vineyards. He was on a quest to harness these polyphenols so they could be put to their maximum use.

We chatted some more and ended up discussing what is known as the French paradox. This was all the rage at the time thanks to a recent episode of *60 Minutes* featuring scientist Serge Renaud (from Professor Vercauteren's alma mater), who had discussed the fact that although the French drink more red wine than practically anyone else (Italians are a distant second!) and consume a diet replete with rich food like cheese, butter, and beef, they nevertheless have the lowest level of cardiovascular disease in the Western world. What could account for it? The answer was all around us: the regular, moderate consumption of red wine. Professor Vercauteren explained that many of the health benefits of the French diet were found in the antioxidant polyphenols in red wine—the very same compound he was studying.

As soon as we heard that, Bertrand and I threw each other a glance. Bertrand had always had an entrepreneurial edge to him, and I had been studying near Grasse with different "noses" (the term for a fragrance expert) in the hopes of pursuing a career in the fragrance and skincare business. The conversation with Professor Vercauteren got us thinking. Here we were, with all these resveratrol-rich grapes at our fingertips—why not explore what polyphenols might be capable of doing for something beauty-related?

So we set up a second meeting with Professor Vercauteren for the very next day. We continued to discuss the French paradox, and he elaborated on his research. He told us that he'd been working on a medication called Endothelon, designed to improve blood circulation, that was made from grape-seed polyphenols and had been doing the scientific work necessary to receive the French equivalent of FDA approval for the drug. He took the research a step further by stabilizing the polyphenols with a fatty acid, making them more bioavailable. Before Professor Vercauteren's patented discoveries, the only way to use polyphenols was to ingest them, but he had figured out a way to use them topically. Not only that, but he was also able to stabilize the polyphenols so that they would stay potent and to patent his process—this patent was vitally important because it was the only way that polyphenols could effectively be used as anti-aging wrinkle fighters in skincare products.

Something about our youthful eagerness and determination must have intrigued this brilliant scientist, because we somehow managed to convince him to work with us. In 1994, Bertrand and I quit the jobs we loved, and from that unassuming day in the sun, a global skincare empire—our life's work, Caudalie—was born.

From day one, I wanted Caudalie to be based on the same principles that surrounded me in the Alpine village of my childhood: the best of nature, eating well and breathing in pure clean air, being comfortable in your own skin as you hiked up a mountain trail, and studying hard to understand the power of science and the world around us. We launched our company in 1995 with two creams and a dietary supplement produced in very small quantities. From these humble roots to today's boutiques and spas, we have worked incredibly hard to build a globally successful business.

I hope you will see *The French Beauty Solution* as the very best of the French attitude toward beauty and skincare filtered through my experiences of learning what American women truly want. I have dedicated my life to discovering and harnessing the most potent ingredients from nature, and this book is infused with that knowledge as well as incredibly useful tips from some of the best beauty scientists, estheticians, and professionals around the world.

HOW TO USE THIS BOOK

This book is divided into five parts. The first is about how your lifestyle affects your beauty, and the remaining four include practical tips so you can easily apply the French beauty philosophy to your daily routine.

Part 1 is loaded with advice on how to live a happy and healthy life the French way. Chapter 1, "The Essence of French Beauty," is an overview of my philosophy and the Pleasure Principle, and in it I discuss iconic French beauties and how we feel about aging with grace. Chapter 2, "Eat Like the French for a Gorgeous Glow," discusses our attitude toward food and explains how what you put in your body affects the outside as well. I eat tasty and nourishing food that energizes instead of drains—and these meals provide just what my skin needs, too. You'll learn not so much what to eat, but *how* to eat, not only to improve your skin from the inside out, but also to gain optimal nutrition without gaining weight. Chapter 3, "Relaxation à la Française," shows you how to recharge yourself while improving your health at the same time. We require a lot of energy to manage everything we need to do—get to work, take care of the kids, run the household—and I know I need to take care of myself if I want to stay healthy and be the best possible mom, wife, and entrepreneur I can be. Have you ever looked at someone who was tired and frazzled and thought, "She's beautiful!" I think *non*.

Part 2 tackles the science behind skincare. Chapter 4, "How Your Skin Ages," gives you the basic facts on how the largest organ of your body works. Chapter 5, "Your Guide to Skincare Ingredients," will teach you which ingredients work, which don't, and which may even be dangerous to your health. This way, you can treat all your skincare concerns without succumbing to false advertising or shelling out money for useless products.

In part 3, I show you how to adopt an effective skincare routine, and I provide recommendations designed to streamline your approach to meet your unique needs. Chapter 6 is about your face and neck, and chapter 7 deals with your body (including hands, feet, and nails) as well as the importance—and luxury—of fragrance. In chapter 8, you'll find a variety of homemade recipes for your skin, many based on treatments that have been tested and are favorites both in our Caudalie spas as well as throughout France.

Chapter 9 in part 4 will teach you everything you need to know about how the French do their makeup, and chapter 10 is devoted to haircare. I share my favorite tips and those of professionals so that you can use makeup to enhance rather than mask your innate beauty, and you'll be able to streamline your hairstyling, too.

Finally, chapter 11 in part 5 shows you how a simple three-day grape detox can be revitalizing and therapeutic. Many people have no idea how to do a cleanse properly and too many are trying to do so in dangerous ways. I teach you how to reap the most benefits with a few days of targeted eating. All the information shared in this book has been tested at our Caudalie Vinotherapie Spas since 1999—and our clients have been enjoying the effects of our Grape Cleanse long before the recent liquid detox craze began.

Et voilà! Let me share my secrets with you!

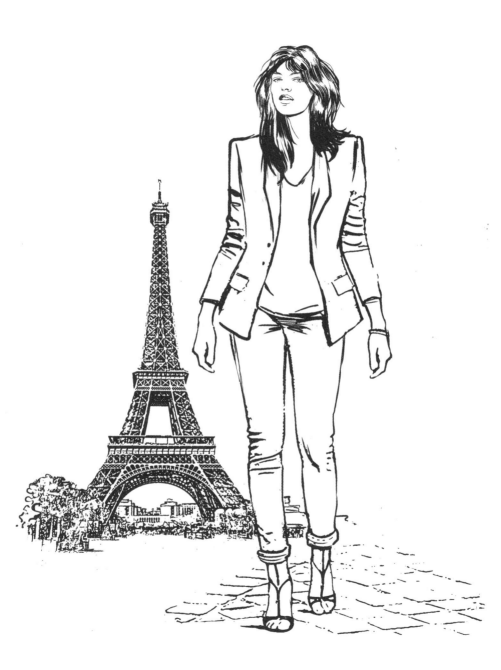

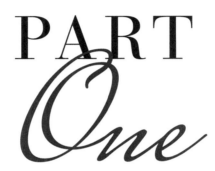

PART One

Lifelong Beauty the French Way

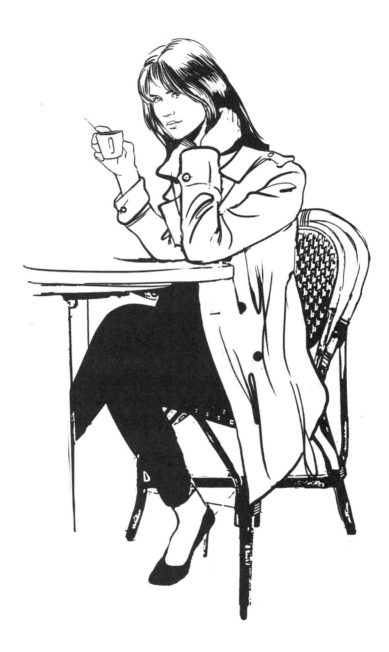

One

THE ESSENCE OF FRENCH BEAUTY

I feel the most beautiful when I'm happy, because only then can
you let go of the fear and just exist in the moment. When people
forget themselves, that's when they are at their most beautiful.

—Juliette Binoche

Ah, the French. Love and light. Fashion and fantasy. Gastronomy
and gamines. Baguettes and Bardot. Perfume and Paris. Sophistication and superiority. Vivaciousness and Versailles. And let us not
forget the guillotine and the Gauloises that will put a swift end to
your romantic romps on the banks of the Seine!

What is it about the French that seemingly leaves American
women envious of our *savoir faire*? What made Edith Wharton
claim that "The French woman is in nearly all respects as different
as possible from the average American woman. The French woman
is more grown-up. Compared with the women of France the aver-

age American woman is still in kindergarten." Even as a proud Frenchwoman, I think Edith was being a little bit harsh. I have spent five years in America and have met thousands of women and can say that American women are often just as sophisticated and grown-up about their beauty and lifestyles as the French are. The difference lies in the way you show it.

Our love for luxe and elegance has always been the hallmark of French style. The nobility may have taxed the lower classes into revolt, with the infamous Marie Antoinette losing her once perfectly coiffed head, but they also were responsible for creating the fashion business and sumptuous style that became the envy of Europe. Compared with the bejeweled and beribboned and bewigged frippery of the French court, our modern-day beauties are positively peasants—but they still strive for that inimitably stylish elegance.

Beauty is an *art de vivre* ("art of living") for Frenchwomen. It is about choosing only the best and understanding that you are entitled to have a beauty routine that makes you look and feel beautiful at the same time. At an early age, we figure out what suits us best, and we set the trends—not follow them. We know that less will always be more, there is no "right" way to be beautiful, and most of all, how you feel about yourself, no matter what your age, is even more important than how you look. It also doesn't hurt that being witty, savvy, smart, and cultured are as essential to beauty as having great skin.

Follow these principles and you'll be like the French in no time at all.

THE ESSENTIALS OF FRENCH BEAUTY
LIVE BY THE PLEASURE PRINCIPLE

The Pleasure Principle is pretty simple. All it means is that your beauty routine should make you *feel* good at the same time it makes you look good.

Luckily, adapting this attitude into your skincare routine is incredibly easy. Once you realize that the best skincare will give you clinically tested and proven results *without* a clinical, medicinal feel, you'll realize that skincare isn't a luxury—but rather that it can and should be *luxurious*, enticing all your senses and making you feel good while it works.

The Pleasure Principle makes it easier for you to make better choices, because you not only have to love what you use but also use what you love. We believe that good skincare isn't about using trendy, hyped, or absurdly expensive products, but about using the most potent and effective ingredients—the ones that have been proven to work for you. We expect them to be deliciously scented, with a texture that feels wonderful on the skin, and with ingredients that are as pure and natural as possible. If it burns or causes redness or smells like something you could shine your car with, then it's not for us. We want all our senses to be effortlessly engaged and believe there should be a palpable pleasure in pampering your skin.

The French have a reputation for being snobbish. But what some may consider arrogance is really an extension of our conviction that we deserve the best. Because we do—and so do you. Americans often believe that the best must also be the most expensive— especially when it comes to beauty products (how many of you bought your first skincare products at the drugstore but, as soon as you had more resources, started shelling out much more for the best products or treatments you could afford?). But for the French, the best does not have to be expensive. Though it's true that high-quality products are often pricier than what you find at the drug-store, there are lots of great products—some of which you can make using ingredients in your kitchen!—that don't have to cost a lot. The best products are those that are best *for you*—what works and what fits with your lifestyle.

The Pleasure Principle is about looking good and feeling good for your own sake—not because it's trendy or to impress other people. This is why we'll wear sexy lingerie underneath a simple button-down shirt and a pair of our favorite jeans. Who cares if no one else will see it? No plain cotton undies for us, *merci beaucoup!*

GOOD SKINCARE IS FAR BETTER
THAN HIDING BEHIND A MASK OF MAKEUP

My beauty routine isn't just about what I put on my skin. It's about all the habits that could have an effect on my skin—diet, environment, sleep, stress, work, travel, and, of course, my family and friends. Before you start to change your products and routines, you have to take a good look at how you treat your body, as it's indeli-bly reflected in the quality of your skin.

For the French, skincare is all about prevention and treat-ment, but, because we follow the Pleasure Principle, it is not a chore. While we'd no more dream of sleeping in our makeup than we would eat our daily lunch at fast-food restaurants, the Pleasure Principle allows us to make the daily necessity of proper skincare as easy and as enticing as possible.

The keyword here is *maintenance*—and you're never too young to start. When we were teenagers, my friends and I were sternly warned by our mothers not to set foot out the door without first applying an antioxidant moisturizer with SPF in the morning and to cleanse our faces particularly well at night. That set us up for a lifetime of a minimal yet effective skincare maintenance because the emphasis was on protecting the skin, not covering up flaws with pore-clogging foundation.

If we had acne, we hastened to the dermatologist and were given a range of treatment options, sometimes including birth control pills once we were sixteen or seventeen (mainly because they were such an effective weapon against pimples). In addition, because *pharmacies* in France are much more personalized than drugstores in America tend to be, with comprehensive skincare centers and pharmacists and other staff well trained in skin issues, we bought our products there and felt confident that they were effective.

My mother was far more obsessed with having shiny hair and smooth skin than she ever was about makeup. She loved to try new antiwrinkle creams, and her bathroom shelves looked like an apothecary, but she rarely used more makeup than a bit of mascara and a neutral lipstick. I followed her example and the first makeup product I ever bought was a super-sheer bronzer, Terracotta by Guerlain. My friends also bought it, and maybe we'd add a sheer lip gloss, a swipe of mascara on our top lashes, and a quick brush through our hair, and we were done.

When I tell this to the American women or their young daughters I meet on my travels, their eyes get wide. "Really?" they say. "That's *it?*" I say yes, but I can tell they don't believe me!

While I use a few more skincare products and my makeup bag is just a bit fuller now, this routine has barely changed two decades later. I started it so early that I prevented a lot of damage to my skin that would have happened otherwise.

LESS IS MORE

Many women think that in order to be as vibrant and remain as youthful as possible, they have to be on an endless starvation diet, shuddering at the mere thought of a slice of bread and sweet cream butter; work out like a fiend with a personal trainer or shred their muscles at CrossFit; swallow twenty-six different supplements every morning; slather on ultra-expensive creams, day and night; and have their cosmetic dermatologist on speed dial as they shell out thousands for lasers or injectable fillers or other painful procedures. Trust me—that is *not* the French way!

When American women tell me that their French counterparts make it "look so easy," I tell them that's because, for us, it is, but only because we streamline our beauty routine and know that less is more. Yes, it's always fun to try some of the crazy new products out there—and because I need to constantly test new products for my business, I am always working on new items—but basically, as you'll see in part 3, it's simple: cleanser, toner, eye cream, serum, and moisturizer with SPF in the morning, and ditto at night (without the SPF and always take off that eye makeup!). Exfoliate at least twice a week to remove dead skin cells. Use masks regularly for treatment and hydration. *Voilà!*

NEVER GO ON A DIET, AND NEVER EAT PROCESSED FOOD

Diets don't work. Chapter 2 tells you how to eat like the French, so all I'll say here is that dieting wreaks havoc not only on your metabolism but also your skin. Who wants to starve and have an ashy and wan complexion at the same time? *Pas moi!* Eating good, real, natural foods consistently—and especially cooking them yourself, so you can ensure that nothing processed, chemical, or artificial is included—and making sure you get the proper nutrients are key to looking good from the inside out. The French pay attention to what they eat . . . and drink. *Vive le French paradox!*

A GLASS OF RED WINE AT DINNER IS
GOOD FOR YOUR SKIN (AND YOUR HEALTH)

You'll learn much more about the power of polyphenols and the other nutrient-laden compounds in red wine in parts 2 and 5 of this book, but suffice it to say here that one glass of red wine sipped slowly with your dinner will not only improve your meal but your health, too. It will also relax you and improve your look, and that will show most noticeably in your skin.

BE COMFORTABLE IN YOUR OWN SKIN

The summer I was thirteen, my parents sent me to a camp in California, not far from Los Angeles, with two of my French friends. After we got settled in and joined the other campers for sunbathing, we, naturally, took off our tops so we wouldn't have to worry about tan lines from our bikinis (what can I tell you—we were still very young and didn't think twice about sun damage!). Needless to say, this was a bit of a disaster, even though it was almost worth seeing the shocked looks of our fellow campers and counselors. I must confess that we had done it just a little bit to see if we could get away with it—but we also did it because we'd always done it. No one in France wears a top at the beach. Casual nudity was absolutely no big deal. It became a big deal only when people in California—the land of golden sunshine and soft sandy beaches so tantalizing to a French girl—tried to shame us. Fortunately, we knew our parents would roll their eyes at the prudish Americans. And they did.

The French definitely do not have the Puritan squeamishness about the human body and its functions that permeates a lot of

American culture. We live in the land of the bidet, remember! And we are constantly amazed at how Americans will yell at a nursing mother to cover up when she tries to breastfeed in public, but have no problem with hypersexualized ads in magazines and on billboards where young women pose in next to nothing in order to sell designer jeans. That attitude has trickled down to my children, who now think that going topless on the beach or at home is "disgusting." When I told my parents that my children referred to my post-shower nakedness as "inappropriate," they howled with laughter. There is, after all, no proper translation in French for "inappropriate nudity" within the family home (or at the beach).

Our bodies, no matter their size, are wonderful creations. We were born nude and take off clothes out of necessity several times a day. I think this is one reason the French make beauty seem so effortless—we are raised to always feel good in our skin.

I think this is one of the reasons American women tend to package themselves and hide behind a mask of makeup. The hair is done just so and the makeup is flawless and the shoes are shiny and the outfit styled and coordinated. But if the woman behind it all is self-conscious, it shows. Beauty radiates from within and cannot be faked. It's painfully obvious when someone is not at ease with herself. She'll surreptitiously check the mirror every few minutes. She'll ask her friends for reassurance. And she'll go to the ladies' room for a good cry if she asks the question, "Does my butt look big in this?" and doesn't get the answer she craves within a nanosecond.

EMBRACE YOUR QUIRKS

Perfection is boring. Frenchwomen don't take ourselves too seriously, and neither should you!

It's much easier to embrace your quirks when you are comfortable in your own skin, as I said above. The French are more accepting of idiosyncratic beauty, even flaunting it, while Americans fixate on the quirk and wonder why it's been played up. Have a nose that's a tad long, or ears that stick out a bit, or brows that are a little crooked, or lips with an unusual shape? Freckles that won't quit? Who cares? They're all fabulous.

Take Brigitte Bardot. She was jaw-droppingly beautiful and had the cutest overbite that made men go mad wishing they could kiss her. Americans looked at her and said, "Oh, yes, she's gorgeous, she's adorable, what a great figure in that white bikini, but did you see those teeth? What an overbite! Why didn't she get them fixed?"

As you'll see in the list of Iconic French Beauties on pages 29 and 38, some of the most celebrated faces in France have a noticeable quirk, like the gap in Vanessa Paradis's front teeth or Charlotte Rampling's hooded eyelids or Charlotte Gainsbourg's near plainness that can quickly morph into beauty, like that of her sister Lou Doillon. We also adore quirky beauty in women from other countries, like androgynous Tilda Swinton, Cindy Crawford and her famous mole, or Anjelica Huston with her amazing Roman nose. It's what makes these women even more memorable.

NEVER LOOK AS IF YOU'RE TRYING TOO HARD

The French love the no-makeup makeup look more than any other. Crave those smoky eyes? *Très bien,* but your lips should be bare. Love that new bloodred lipstick? *Très bien,* but your eyes should have nothing more than a hint of mascara.

Parisian women putting on their makeup are seemingly like ducks on a pond, gliding with ease. They make it look so effortless. What you don't see, of course, is the effort that went into that effortlessness, just as you don't see the duck's webbed feet furiously paddling under water. And when you tell your French friends that their faces look amazing, they'll say, "Oh, yes. But I did nothing, really. It's so quick and easy. Just a bit of this and that, and *voilà!*"

In other words, the no-makeup makeup look does take time to master at first. That's the key—*at first*. (Don't worry—you'll learn exactly what to do in chapter 9).

Strive for a calculated nonchalance in your behavior (no waiting by the phone for him to call, *merci beaucoup!*) and in your makeup and hairstyling. You'll look French in no time at all. And you can finally throw away all those unused tubes and containers you know you'll never use again.

THERE'S ALWAYS ANOTHER LIPSTICK

Although the French are secure in what looks best on them, they're always willing to try a new color or texture—and just as willing to chuck it if it doesn't work. In other words, even the French, who adore the no-makeup makeup look, don't want to get stuck in a beauty rut. Be adventurous within the parameters of what you know looks best on you.

And when you're in the mood to be adventurous, do what my friend Delphine Sicard, a celebrated makeup artist, said: "*Bien sur,* you should experiment with new stuff, but don't be adventurous with boys. Be adventurous with your girlfriends first and ask them what they think. Then try it out on the boys and see what happens!"

NO PAIN, NO GAIN, NO WAY!

That great beauty demands great suffering is a concept guaranteed to make the French say, "*La vie est trop courte.*" Life is too short.

I think Americans are willing to undergo treatments that are very painful or too harsh because they think it makes them look better. The French believe that if a beauty treatment is painful, if the product stings, if something doesn't feel right, if everyone says it's the only way to go, it's not a good thing to do, and we won't do it!

NEVER GO TO BED WITH YOUR MAKEUP STILL ON

Even if you've been up drinking Champagne with your lover all night, you *will* take off your makeup and wash your face, and you *will* hydrate it afterward. Your French *maman* would not be shocked by how much Champagne you drank—but she would be horrified if you fell asleep with your mascara on.

SQUEAKY CLEAN IS FOR WINDOWS—NOT YOUR FACE OR HAIR

Many American women I've met told me that they were always instructed to wash their hair until it was *squeaky* clean. They'd lather, rinse, and repeat, and then wonder why their hair was so dry and damaged. Or they'd scrub their face until it was practically raw in an effort to catch every bit of dirt or oil that lingered. This is not only the antithesis of the Pleasure Principle, but it also strips off the natural oils that give hair its shine and give skin a vibrant texture. Go for the gentle to get the glow.

BEAUTY DOESN'T END AT YOUR CHIN

The French consider the face to include everything that extends from the tip of your head down to your décolleté. That means you treat your neck and décolleté exactly as and when you treat your face. Don't forget the rest of you, too! Read lots more about this in chapter 7.

PROFESSIONAL BEAUTY TREATMENTS ARE
A NECESSITY, NOT A LUXURY

I discuss this at length in chapter 3, but we know that whatever a good, professional treatment costs is well worth it in superior results. We don't consider regular facials to be a luxurious treat we'd indulge in maybe once a year. They're a necessary part of our regular skincare regimen, and as there's a cumulative effect from good treatments and the use of good products, that encourages us to keep up with this maintenance. Fortunately, treatments at salons or day spas are far less expensive in France (even in Paris) than they tend to be in America—probably because we go so often that the price can stay affordable. (Americans, on the other hand, have fantastically inexpensive nail salons, so you go for regular manicures while the French tend to do it themselves.)

According to my friend Dr. Bernard Hertzog, a cosmetic physician beloved by the beautiful ladies of Paris and London for his subtle ways with complexion-brightening mesotherapy that restore fullness to thinning faces, "Frenchwomen with no particular skin issues regularly get advice from their esthetician or a trained pharmacist who sells cosmetic products. Their approach is usually the same: Moisturize the skin and protect it from the sun, since UV rays' harmful effects on the skin are more and more taken seriously in France and Europe.

"The bigger the skin issue is, the more medical its approach will be," he adds. "When the skin issue is persistent or gets worse, they will consult a dermatologist. In that case, we are not in the cosmetic field anymore, but the medical one, where the purpose is more therapeutic than cosmetic."

Listen to Bernard and don't treat your skincare as if it's superfluous. Do you go to the dentist twice a year to make sure your teeth are clean and healthy? Why wouldn't you give the same consideration to your skin?

IT'S NOT A RACE

As you'll see in chapter 3, the French are much better at downtime and realizing that life may be short but it's a not a sprint to the finish line. We don't want to burn out because we feel the pressure, as so many American women do, to have babies and go to kickboxing class and have a high-pressure career and send their children to the "right" preschool. We look at that pressure with much sympathy and are grateful for our *joie de vivre* and long vacations—we know what all that stress does to our skin. I see that every day in New York. This is a truly wonderful city for working, but Paris is a truly wonderful city for *living*.

HAVE A LOVER WHO LOVES YOUR BODY (AND THE REST OF YOU)

French teenagers can sometimes be very naughty. We used to tease each other by saying, "The reason you get zits is because you don't have a lover!" Mind you, we weren't exactly ready for lovers when we were teenagers with zits.

But we did know that, when we grew up, making love was guaranteed to improve our complexion, giving our cheeks that unique rosy glow.

BEAUTY DOES NOT MEAN ONLY YOUTH

It's always a bit of a shock for me when I go back to France and see my longtime friends. They're around my age and they're still very beautiful—and they have the wrinkles that naturally come with being a woman in your forties. I don't see that so much anymore in New York City, where women of a certain age have unnaturally plumped up their faces in an effort to get rid of any wrinkle or blemish that could signal how old they are.

But I think my best friends look *better* because they look like themselves. I know they're never going to get to the point where their faces are totally smooth and plastic and the rest of them isn't—they know, as I do, that as soon as you remove wrinkles from one area, they're going to sprout somewhere else! The only thing that ever truly works is to protect yourself from the sun, stay hydrated with the best possible skincare products, and follow the tips in this book. That's a lot easier than worrying over every new line that appears overnight.

Wrinkles are a sign that you've *lived,* and laugh lines are called that for a reason. Cherish the memories of your plump young cheeks and embrace the stunning cheekbones you have now. Confidence in your appearance and an air of contentment makes even an octogenarian look decades younger than a hipster trying too hard to be chic.

This reminds me of a little story an American friend recently told me: "I was in Paris for the first time and my boyfriend and I were having lunch at a small outdoor café on a warm summer's day," she said. "A Frenchwoman, probably in her late sixties or early seventies, sat down at a table next to ours. Obviously, Paris is great for people-watching, but I was particularly struck by her, as she was dressed better than most of the Frenchwomen I'd seen that week; better, in fact, than most people I encounter on a regular basis—and I live in New York City! She was wearing a light sweater with a nautical pattern and that fit her perfectly, impeccably tailored khaki capris, saddle shoes, and a scarf—nothing fancy, but it suited her perfectly. And the shoes! They were bright orange—not an obnoxious orange but kind of a burnt orange. Very eye-catching but very classy. She just absolutely radiated style and chic.

"What struck me the most was that she looked amazing, but she also looked her age. She was dressed fashionably but she wasn't trying to be too youthful. Her hair was a subtle silver, and not dyed an obvious color as a New Yorker of the same age would likely do. Unlike many Americans I know or have seen, she wasn't trying too hard by wearing too-tight or ultra-trendy clothes; nor had she given up, embracing pants with elastic waistbands and dowdy tops. I realized that for the French, beauty is something that changes with age. What is beautiful at twenty is wholly different from what is beautiful at forty or sixty or beyond. The difference is, it's still beautiful. When I looked at this woman, I didn't think, 'Oh, she looks good for her age.' I thought, 'She looks good. Period.'"

This lovely Frenchwoman knew that style is everything when you age. You don't want to look too bourgeois with hair too perfectly coiffed or too much masklike makeup on. A little bit of rock 'n' roll attitude is a good thing.

Aging with grace means finding that healthy balance of your work life, family life, love life, and inner life, too. Coco Chanel once said, "As you get older, you get the face you deserve." I don't think she meant this in the nicest possible way, but I do think that if you're always stressed or angry or frustrated, or if you hold on to what happened in the past and let that define your future, a certain hardness will creep into your features that will not make you look happy or the best you possibly can.

Also, if you focus solely on having a smooth complexion, you're not only going to look older, but you're also not going to be a very interesting person. After all, your appearance is only one aspect of what makes you unique, and uniquely beautiful. The more interests you have in life, the more interesting, curious, engaged, and sparkling you become.

The French attitude about aging is that it's inevitable. You can fight it like the uber-ambitious women I see every day in New York. For them, aging is war and they are going to do whatever it takes to win every battle.

But the French know it's a fight that can't ever be won, because time never tires of marching on. Instead of fighting the inevitability of aging, we're going to embrace it. We're going to do what we can. We're going to try to have a balanced life, to not just focus on our faces but on *all* the faces in our lives. We're going to try to be generous and do the best we can, in every realm that's important to us. Most of all, we're going to live in the here and now—not the nebulous, unpredictable future—so we can be happy with what we've got and not what we'll never have.

And we'll always wash our faces every night!

ICONIC FRENCH BEAUTIES OVER FIFTY
(AND BELIEVE ME, THAT IS *NOT* OLD!)

BRIGITTE BARDOT

"What could be more beautiful than a dear old lady growing wise with age? Every age can be enchanting, provided you live with it."

Blessed with the sexiest overbite ever, Brigitte (or BB, as the French loved to call her) was trained as a ballerina, giving her an openness with her body that had rarely been seen before. That she was beautifully proportioned and had an astonishing mass of thick blond hair didn't hurt, either. Her iconic cat's-eye makeup and red lipstick have never gone out of style, but she has also unwittingly become the poster child for the effects of sun damage and heavy smoking on a woman's skin. Back when she was rocking a bikini, sunscreen was barely used by consumers and women slathered on baby oil and baked themselves to get that Saint-Tropez tan. So her face may be heavily lined, but she is still BB and still a beauty.

JULIETTE BINOCHE

"Fighting the aging process just doesn't work. I think that actresses, ultimately, are responsible for the faces we give to women. But I understand the fear, you know? I really do: It's easy to think 'I'll never work again if I lose some of my beauty.'... The thing is that I never felt beautiful. I think I can change my looks and be different things, but I've never thought of myself as this face."

Juliette positively radiates intelligence. She never wears a lot of makeup—she doesn't need to. She does change her hairstyles quite a lot and looks equally good with short hair and bangs and with longer locks. She is a dazzling example of being at ease in her own skin. We were so happy when she was the godmother of our annual harvest festival at Château Smith Haut Lafitte in Bordeaux, Les Accabailles, one year, too.

CAROLE BOUQUET

"I was very shy. Being considered beautiful, I always felt that people were waiting for something more. I imagined you were supposed to have an intellectual ability—and I'm making no claims here—proportional to your supposed good looks . . . I felt I should be proving I deserved the attention; that I should be doing something special."

A former face of Chanel and well-known as one of the James Bond girls, Carole is the essence of Parisian chic, with perfectly symmetrical features. Her hair is always done simply and she doesn't wear a lot of makeup—she didn't even as a Chanel model. She is just classy and is aging beautifully with grace and style.

CATHERINE DENEUVE

"The way a woman ages has much to do with genetics. My mother has very good bone structure, which I have inherited, and it certainly helps. My mother also gave me my two most important beauty tips—to be careful of the sun and to drink lots of water."

There is a now-classic saying attributed to Catherine that goes something like this: "After the age of forty, a woman must choose between her ass and her face." Meaning that as you grow older and the skin of your face loses its youthful contours, a bit of padding helps minimize wrinkles—but if your body is too thin, you'll look gaunt and haggard. Funnily enough, Catherine has often claimed she never said that, but in any case, her posterior is still quite lovely and her face even more so. She may have had a bit of work done and she may not be as svelte as she was in *Belle de Jour*, but she is still ravishingly beautiful.

ISABELLE HUPPERT

"I never really behaved as a beautiful person, even as a young adult. I never really trusted myself in that respect, but then when I look back, I think, 'Oh, after all, I was okay.'"

You don't normally see a lot of freckles on French skin, but then again you don't see a lot of women who look like Isabelle, either. Even though she has an air of impenetrability, which makes her one of France's most accomplished actresses, you can't take your eyes off her. Especially when she wears almost no makeup except a bright, matte red lipstick. Less is more!

CHARLOTTE RAMPLING

"I have boxes of pictures of myself and have many of them framed. I'm always surprised to see that I looked like that."

What a perfect choice, at age sixty-eight, for the NARS makeup campaign in the fall of 2014. "She is a natural beauty that feels strong, yet relatable," François Nars himself told *Women's Wear Daily*. Charlotte has an unusually masculine bone structure and deep-set eyes, giving her a naturally strong and fearless (and super-sexy) look. She is unabashed about the wrinkles that come with age, and I wish that more women followed her example because she is modern, rock 'n' roll, and not too bourgeois.

WHAT MAKES YOU LOOK OLD

There are many things you might be inadvertently doing that add years to your appearance. Frenchwomen try their utmost to avoid what's on this list:

- Foundation that's too thick, too obvious, or that isn't blended well. Having your face be a different tone from your neck or the rest of your body is a definite *non*.

- A super-matte, powdered face.

- Too much blush, or blush that isn't the right (subtle) color.

- Eyebrows that are too thin or the wrong shape for your face.

- Creamy eye shadow that tends to crease in your lids as the day goes on.

- Too much mascara, mainly because your lashes tend to thin out as you age. Avoid super-black and go for a more natural brown-black. Apply it only to the bottom part of your lashes instead of extending it all the way to the tips, and also avoid putting any mascara on your lower lashes.

- Neon or super-bright colors. Soften your palette as you get older.

- Lip liner that is obvious, especially if it's darker than your lipstick.

- Super-shiny lip gloss.

- Borrowing your daughter's lipstick (or anything else in her makeup bag, as well as in her closet—particularly her leather miniskirt).

- Yellow teeth.

- Gray hair that is not beautifully styled—lots of women look stunning with salt-and-pepper or silver or white hair, but once your hair color is gone, evening out the tone is crucial.

- The same haircut you've had for decades.

- The same hair color you've had for decades. When you get older, go softer and lighter.

- Not eating well. When you starve yourself into thinness, it shows on your face. Or when you deprive yourself of delicious food, it makes you feel and look pinched.

- Not getting enough sleep.

- Too much stress.

- Not being dynamic. Being out of shape is an instant ager.

- Not being curious. Being interested in the world makes you look and feel young.

- Not being open-minded. You know by now that the French aren't as prudish as the Americans. We love our bodies and we love sex and we love talking about it. In addition, we're part of Europe, and all we have to do is drive for a few hours to be in a different country where everything is different. It helps keep us adventurous.

- Not challenging yourself. You can never, ever give up on life—or your appearance. Giving up instantly makes you look old. So you tried that diet and it didn't work (because diets don't work, no matter how much you stick to them)? Don't just say, "Oh, I'm so fat, I'm never going to get it right. It's not worth it." Instead, say, "From now on, I'm going to eat like the French. I'm going to make the most delicious meals ever—just with smaller portions—and I'm going to savor every morsel, and I am going to lose weight and enjoy myself while the pounds are disappearing." That is the kind of attitude that will immediately make you look and feel ten years younger.

- Forgoing that glass of red wine with dinner.

WHAT THE FRENCH ENVY ABOUT THE AMERICANS

Believe it or not, there are many things about America and Americans that Frenchwomen envy:

- Your beautiful breasts that always seem to be more shapely than ours, even if they really aren't!

- Your sparkling white, straight teeth, thanks to years of fluoride-rich water and good dentistry and orthodontia.

- Your strong muscles and bones. Perhaps it's the milk and meat and corn you tend to eat as part of your regular diet when growing up, but American women tend to look so much more fit and healthy than the French. Super-sporty cheerleaders and runners and gym-goers are always a source of awe.

- Your amazing models. When I was a teenager, the top American models were Cindy Crawford, Christy Turlington, Janice

Dickinson, Stephanie Seymour, and Christie Brinkley. That hair, that skin, those glamazon legs, those powerful yet slim and shapely bodies! They exuded vibrant health and glamour without even trying.

- Your amazing nails. The colors, the textures, the shapes. Our manicures and pedicures are very boring in comparison.

- Your discipline when it comes to bad habits. Frenchwomen tend to smoke way too much. They know it's a terrible, life-threatening habit, and they don't beat themselves up about it—when they should. Americans can go to the other extreme of "Oh my god, I'm going to get cancer if I have one ciga-rette," or "I'm an alcoholic if I have one glass of wine." That attitude will automatically make us want to light up and then order a bottle of Champagne.

- Your boundless energy. We just love America, and especially New York. Even though the city has been cleaned up in recent years, forcing out many of the artists and creative talent that gave New York its edge, there is still a special vibe and it is full of creative and ambitious people doing things to change the world. And, of course, Americans all over the country contin-ually impress me with their innovation, ambition, gumption, and smarts, too.

- Your innovation. American beauty companies are extremely competitive and always looking to launch the next big trend. Whatever they decide to release—whether it's new peels, dy-namic masks, or oils for cleaning your skin (a concept that took a while for Americans to understand, even though these products are incredibly good for your complexion)—will reso-nate all over the world. The raw ingredients may be sourced from other countries, but the know-how to get these products out onto shelves is thanks to the genius of American sales-manship and marketing.

- Your in-your-face humor. The French aren't very good at laughing at themselves. We can take ourselves *way* too seriously. I love seeing laugh lines on a woman because I know that whoever has them loves to find joy in everything she can.

- Your willingness to tell all. In America, what you see is what you get; in Paris it takes way more time to break the eggshell around a person. We excel at keeping secrets, and that's not always a good thing. Not being able to talk about how you feel is often incredibly stressful, and eventually that stress is going to make itself visible in your complexion—and every other aspect of your life.

- Your complaining actually gets you somewhere. The French excel at complaining—but we often complain and then throw up our hands without accomplishing anything. If you, on the other hand, buy a new moisturizer and it doesn't work as promised, you don't hesitate to take it back and demand a refund. Because you know you'll get one.

- Your drive to succeed. The French can get a bit lazy, as sometimes they want to be happy rather than successful.

- In America, anything is possible. French society is much more closed-off and caste driven (even if we claim it's not). In France, who you are and where you were born defines many aspects of your life. In America, you can come from anywhere and end up on top. You can redefine yourself and start all over again and no one will bat an eyelash—in fact, they'll encourage you to go for it.

Just don't get stuck in a beauty rut on your way to success!

ICONIC FRENCH BEAUTIES UNDER FIFTY

MARION COTILLARD

"I'm never really aware [of my looks] because I'm not very interested in it. I don't need it."

Marion lives a quiet and simple life with her family near Bordeaux (where she likes to come to the Caudalie spa). She is passionate about using only the most natural and organic products on her skin—and it shows. She's even more beautiful because she's smart and stays true to her values and what she believes in. I can attest to the fact that she has the most perfect naked skin I've ever seen.

CHARLOTTE GAINSBOURG

"My mother is a great example of someone who has done nothing, although she was born very beautiful. She said that during the 1960s, due to all the makeup, all the girls looked the same. She said you should stay as authentic as possible."

Daughter of French icon and singer Serge Gainsbourg and fashion icon Jane Birkin, Charlotte has always been extremely slim, and has that wonderful edginess that makes her so effortlessly stylish. She is a nonconformist beauty, who can play the plain Jane and then tilt her head and become extremely beautiful—which is why she was perfectly cast as the eponymous heroine in one of the film versions of *Jane Eyre*.

EVA GREEN

"Everything is in the eyes. The soul is in the eyes, and it makes it sharper. I wear no makeup in real life. I'm very simple. That may be why I go over the top for the red carpet. But otherwise, I'm very plain. I should make more of an effort, actually."

Overtly sexual and sensual in her performances, Eva Green has a perfect pout and knows how to flaunt it. Of all the French beauties, she is the most American inasmuch as she tends to hide behind a mask of makeup—but only when she knows she'll be in the public eye. It's interesting to see her in photos with her twin sister; you can tell which one is the star who has a certain image to uphold.

SOPHIE MARCEAU

"I've never really been beautiful. I'm photogenic, which is very important, and now I'm getting older I'm aware I have to take care."

For me, Sophie is the epitome of a woman in her forties who is, of course, no longer very young but is still more than youthful in spirit. She's the French equivalent of the stunning girl next door, a sort of Gallic version of Jennifer Aniston. I think she looks even better now than she did when she was starring in *Braveheart*. And she's especially popular in Asia, where many women think of her as the epitome of French beauty.

VANESSA PARADIS

"Why would I fix [my teeth]? I was born with them. I can spit water through them. They're useful!"

The ageless gamine, Vanessa is a seamless blend of punk and hippie meets Chanel. She rarely wears makeup and the gap between her front teeth (called *les dents du bonheur*, or "lucky teeth") only makes her more endearing. She is such a lovely person and happily admits that she is a lover of wine and beauty treatments. If you look at a lot of photos, you'll see that taking care of her hair is low on her priority list—but she still manages to make bed head look stylish.

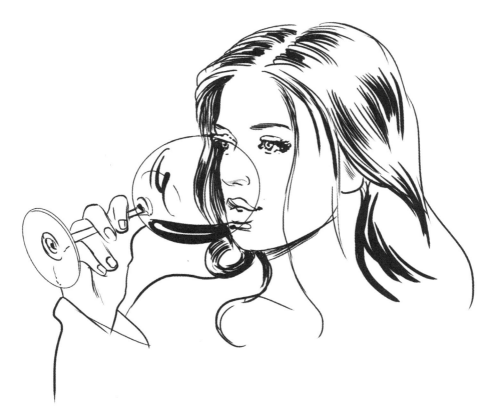

Two

EAT LIKE THE FRENCH FOR A GORGEOUS GLOW

*I could never have been a model in the way actresses today are
expected to be; I was never thin enough. I love a wonderful meal
at the end of the day and a good Bordeaux. I try to be careful but
I am not American—I am not always worrying about calories
and working out.*

—Catherine Deneuve

Good skincare starts the moment you wake up in the morning—
with what you eat and drink. Ideally, a balanced diet full of
antioxidant-laden vegetables and fruits, with only minimal amounts
of processed or junk food, will give you the healthiest possible skin.

The typical French diet follows the guidelines of the
Mediterranean-type diet: fresh vegetables and fruit, whole grains,
nuts, legumes, olive oil, and fish, with some dairy, little meat, and
even less processed food. A study called "Nutritional Skin Care:

Health Effects of Micronutrients and Fatty Acids," published in the *American Journal of Clinical Nutrition* in May 2001, supported the finding that eating a Mediterannean-type diet will make you live longer. What's most important about this kind of eating is that these wholesome foods are not just powerhouses of nutrition but are loaded with omega-3 and omega-6 essential fatty acids, which are needed to keep your cell membranes healthy. And these foods are loaded with antioxidants, too—which you'll read much more about in part 2.

Because your skin is the largest organ in your body, it reflects what's put into it when you eat—and not just what you eat, but *how* you eat. When you drink lots of good mineral water and tea and stay away from junk, your digestive system works as it should, and you glow (being constipated definitely has an unfortunate effect on your skin). When you eat enough of the good fats your body needs for energy and to produce the oils that make your skin look healthy, you glow. When you don't go on starvation diets that make you feel and look pinched, you glow.

Read on, and I'll show you *what* to eat and *how* to eat for optimum skin health.

THE BEST FOODS TO EAT FOR YOUR SKIN

For the healthiest skin, you should eat food high in two categories: antioxidant and essential fatty acids (EFAs).

ANTIOXIDANT FOODS

You'll learn much more about this in chapter 4, but for now, all you need to know is that when your body uses oxygen, cells naturally form by-products called free radicals, which can damage cells and contribute to and accelerate the aging process. Antioxidants neutralize free radicals, which is why they need to be a regular part of your diet and skincare regimen.

According to the Human Nutrition Research Center on Aging at Tufts University, the fruits with the highest antioxidant levels are wild blueberries, blackberries, raspberries, strawberries, prunes, plums, raisins, red grapes, oranges, and cherries. The highest levels in vegetables are found in kale, spinach, Brussels sprouts, alfalfa sprouts, broccoli florets, and beets.

Vitamins A, C, and E are the antioxidant vitamins and selenium a mineral; lycopene is an antioxidant compound that is especially good for your blood vessels; and polyphenols are powerhouse antioxidants that you'll read about in depth in chapter 4. Choose these foods for high antioxidant levels:

- Vitamin A/beta-carotene
  Broccoli, cantaloupe, carrots, egg yolks, fortified grains, fortified milk, liver, low-fat dairy products, mangoes, peaches, pumpkin, squash, tomatoes, yams

- Vitamin C
  Broccoli, cantaloupe, citrus fruits and juices, collard greens, green peppers, kale, kiwi, papaya, parsley, raw cabbage, spinach, strawberries

- Vitamin E
  Broccoli, dried apricots, fish, fish oils, fortified cereals, nuts, seeds, shrimp, vegetable oils, whole grains

- Lycopene
  Tomatoes

- Polyphenols

  Grapes (especially red and especially the skin and seeds), red wine, all berries, goji berries

- Selenium

  Eggs, garlic, seafood, whole-grain cereals

EFA FOODS

Another important nutrient for your skin are the EFAs, particularly omega-3 and omega-6. They play an important role in the regulation of your immune system, lessen inflammation, and also have a skin barrier function. EFAs can be a tremendous help if you have dry skin, reactive and sensitive skin, eczema, or skin irritations. They're also particularly good when the seasons change or before sun exposure.

The best sources of EFAs are cold-water fish like salmon, herring, and mackerel; olive oil and grape-seed oil; walnuts and almonds; dark green leafy vegetables; whole-grain foods; and eggs.

HOW MUCH WATER DO YOU NEED TO DRINK FOR HEALTHY SKIN?

The French were drinking bottled water long before it became ubiquitous in America—not just for its portability but for its mineral content. Unlike most American bottled water, which often isn't even spring water, French water from natural springs is full of useful minerals that help the body absorb nutrients while also hydrating you. The most common minerals found in these waters are calcium, magnesium, potassium, and sodium. All French *marchés* and supermarkets have extensive sections for various waters, and each brand has a different taste and composition depending on where it's sourced; some are also naturally carbonated. Perrier, for example, is very low in sodium and Vichy water very high, while Apollinaris is high in magnesium. I like Vichy Célestins and Hépar brands for glowing skin, but I hesitate to endorse any plastic water bottles when recycling is so important. I have water filters installed in all the Caudalie offices around the world as well as in our spas, which is good for everyone and for the environment, too, and I drink filtered water and my favorite caffeine-free Rooibos or Caudalie draining organic herbal teas all day so I know I'm staying hydrated. This habit also keeps my appetite down as drinks help make your stomach feel full.

According to the Mayo Clinic, the average person needs approximately eight glasses of water every day—that's sixty-four ounces. The water in your coffee or tea counts toward this figure, as does the water content of your food. If you eat a diet high in watermelon and spinach, for example, which have an abundance of water (which is why they're so low-calorie), you'll be ingesting a lot of water. If you exercise or sweat a lot, are pregnant, or have other health conditions, or if it's hot outside, you need more fluids.

Water is necessary for all bodily functions, and

thirst is your body's signal for it that should never be ignored. If you're severely dehydrated, which can be lethal, your skin will seem to shrink and get wrinkled, but that will change as soon as your body gets the fluids it needs. Normal water intake can't plump your skin to decrease wrinkles, but you still need to drink your eight glasses every day to ensure the health of all your organs, especially your skin.

DO YOU NEED TO TAKE SUPPLEMENTS TO HAVE HEALTHY SKIN?

There is no magic pill or vitamin for skin health. If you eat like the French, you are likely getting the nutrients you need, especially if you regularly consume food high in antioxidants and EFAs. While our bodies must have the RDA (recommended daily allowance) for most vitamins and minerals so that our metabolisms work as efficiently as possible, true deficiencies are rare. That's because Americans tend to eat a lot, especially processed food, and these foods have been supplemented with different vitamins and minerals.

Taking lots of vitamin or mineral supplements might seem like a good idea, but it worries me that American women tend to self-diagnose and go for the pills much more than Frenchwomen do—we'd rather cook up a delicious soup with kale, leeks, onions, potatoes, and garlic that will not only satiate our appetites but give us lots of nutrients that are easily assimilated by our digestive systems. Never take mega-doses of any supplement without checking with your physician first. This is important, as some vitamins like A and E are fat-soluble, meaning they stay in your body, whereas any excess vitamin like C is excreted in your urine. Have your iron and vitamin D levels checked regularly by your physician, as many women are lacking in both, which can cause serious health problems. If your skin suddenly becomes very dry, and you don't think that it's due to environmental changes, such as dry heat in winter or other irritants, it can be an indication of diabetes, hormonal changes, or a thyroid condition and warrants prompt medical attention.

If you do want to take supplements:

- Do not self-diagnose or self-treat! Always discuss any supplementation with your physician. A simple blood test can check your vitamin and mineral levels.

- Peer-reviewed scientific studies reported in the journal *Free Radical Biology & Medicine* in the last two decades have shown that the levels of vitamin E and beta-carotene in your skin decrease after sun exposure. This means that as the antioxidant levels in your skin are depleted, they need to be replaced in order to prevent your skin from aging. For this, you need antioxidant-rich fruits and vegetables, especially those with polyphenols, to replenish levels of vitamins C, E, and beta-carotene from the inside.

- A basic one-a-day multivitamin/mineral supplement for women is usually a good idea for chronic dieters, if only to ensure that you get enough calcium and iron.

- A good probiotic will keep the beneficial bacteria in your intestine flourishing.

- Some women like to take biotin for stronger nails or hair, although few people actually lack normal levels; if you do, be aware that it can take from two to six months before you'll see results.

- If you want to take an EFA supplement, the best sources are virgin vegetable oils (borage oil, primrose oil, grape-seed oils) and fish oils.

THE BEST WAY TO EAT FOR YOUR SKIN

My grandmother was famous for the homemade preserves she made from the wild raspberries we'd pick in the forest every summer. I didn't realize then how lucky I was to have lived on that farm where nearly everything we ate was fresh from our garden or the local *marché* and full of nutrients and flavor. I was even luckier that the farmer next door grew the most fabulous leeks. Oh, how my grandmother craved them! She'd go to our local village every morning for a fresh baguette and other goodies, and when the leeks were in season, she'd pick up a small lemon cake at the *boulangerie* for this farmer—and they'd trade. He got the lemon cake and we got the fabulous leeks. In the winter, when he took extra care to grow even more leeks in his greenhouse, my grandmother had to give him *two* cakes in exchange!

That my grandmother preferred leeks to cake is just one example of how she instilled in us a deep understanding of what it truly meant to enjoy and appreciate a "treat."

I'm sure you've read that some French, even Parisians, have started to succumb, like citizens of so many other countries, to a diet filled with fast, packaged food—even factory-made baguettes (what a sacrilege!)—and all the attendant health issues that can come with a diet that relies on preservatives and junk. But the French, as a nation, still have a much more sacred attitude toward nourishment. For us, eating right isn't just about good food, but about the importance of mealtimes (yes, they are a family affair), not depriving yourself of delicious things to eat, and always striving for balance.

In other words, Frenchwomen like creamery butter slathered on a fresh-from-the-bakery baguette (saturated fat and white flour, *mon Dieu!*) and *café au lait* (hold the soy milk, please). We don't think gluten is the devil. We like stinky ripe cheeses oozing off the plate and a rare steak with a few frites on the side.

And when I tell my American customers how much I love to eat, that I don't deprive myself of anything, and that I have a glass of my family's Bordeaux at dinner every night, sometimes they look at me as if I've sprouted six heads. How can I love food so much yet stay slim? How can I drink every night and not become an alcoholic?

The answer is simple: The essence of eating like the French is to eat very well, but in moderation. No one food can keep you looking young, but eating a well-balanced diet will help you maintain a stable, healthy weight without resorting to crash or fad diets. Besides, delectable, flavor-saturated food is very satiating. So is fresh food, loaded with nutrients and fiber that fill you up quickly. So are "fatty" foods like cheese and butter. Eating savory food this way makes the French disinclined to snack between meals. It also allows us to have much less of a taste for or cravings for sugar, which many recent studies have shown is far more responsible for weight gain than much-maligned fat. After all, what replaces the fat in fat-free foods? Sugar, of course! Other studies have shown that processed foods are one of the biggest causes of obesity because our bodies don't know how to metabolize all those preservatives and chemicals. Again, natural and real is best.

The excellent skincare tips you'll read about in the rest of this book show you how to take care of your beauty from the outside in. Following my suggestions for *how* to eat as the French do will allow you to enhance your beauty regimen from the inside out.

DIETS AND DEPRIVATION NEVER WORK

Diets don't work. They don't work for your weight-loss goals and they wreak havoc on your skin. In fact, they often cause more harm than good.

I've discussed countless diets with my customers, especially when I travel around America, and I am always shocked at how regimented and terribly difficult so many of them are to follow. A highly restrictive diet may work for the very short term and can be fine if you need to lose a few pounds for a special event—when we want to do that very quickly, we stick to the PP/PS plan (*pas de pain/pas de sucre*, or no bread/no sugar), but only for a few days. We know that eating a super-structured, do-not-deviate, you-must-suffer diet that restricts what you eat to a few tasteless things is a recipe for disaster. I love broccoli, but I certainly don't want to eat it with a piece of broiled chicken and nothing else for dinner. This makes no sense to the French because deprivation so often leads to bingeing, and all those days or weeks of suffering can be undone in one evening of raiding the ice cream shelves in the supermarket.

Furthermore, when you restrict calories, your body goes into starvation mode, meaning that it actually needs *fewer* calories to run its metabolism, so you'll pack on the pounds and then some as soon as normal calorie intake is restored.

My philosophy is that if you are craving a piece of chocolate, buy the best possible chocolate you can afford and eat a small piece of it. (Note: I did not say the entire chocolate bar.) Savor it and enjoy every morsel. Do not berate yourself for this little indulgence.

One of the chefs at the Caudalie Spa in Bordeaux has a saying: Eat when it's worth it. If you start eating a cookie and the cookie's not very tasty, why would you want to keep eating it? The

French who go out for a special meal at a *gastronomique* restaurant might consume 2,500–3,000 calories in one meal—but they don't beat themselves up over it. They talk about how delicious it was, how it was worth the trip, and then make sure to skip breakfast and not overdo it the next day.

Punishing yourself over food is counterproductive and the exact opposite of what the Pleasure Principle is all about. I hear my American friends say things like, "I know I shouldn't, I really shouldn't, okay I will," driving themselves crazy over a few spoonfuls of dessert. And then they add, "I can't believe I did that, I'm so bad, I'm horrible. I'm such a pig. I'm going on a diet tomorrow." *C'est de la folie!* That's crazy!

Next time you're tempted to jump on the latest fad diet bandwagon, remember that constant weight fluctuation can have an unfortunate effect on your skin. This is an important point if you're a yo-yo dieter. Think about it: If your face expands, then shrinks, then expands and shrinks again with your weight changes, over time your skin will stretch and lose its elasticity. As you get older, it just doesn't bounce back as easily. I'll discuss this at length in part 2.

EAT REAL FOOD, ESPECIALLY VEGETABLES

Packaged foods are anathema to the Frenchwomen I know. We go to the local *marchés* at lunchtime or after work and buy whatever looks fresh and delectable, and then we make a simple meal. I have an American friend who rented a house in the Dordogne Province one summer, and she told me that her friends and family staying with her ate and ate and ate, yet they all lost weight. They walked to the nearby village for a fresh baguette and *café* in the morning, then went out exploring. They didn't snack. They tried all the local delicacies. They drank red wine with dinner. They lost weight without even trying because they were eating the French way—good, real, fresh, super-tasty, local food, eaten with pleasure.

It's easier to eat real food when you don't buy junk in the first place. I was astonished when I moved to New York City and went to the supermarket and saw what was targeted toward children. Prepackaged "lunches" with deli-type meat laden with preservatives, chemicals, and sodium; crackers made with high-fructose corn syrup guaranteed to send their blood sugar soaring; and a sweetened drink that was nothing but more high-fructose corn syrup and food coloring. And then there's pasta with tomato sauce in a can, or a vinaigrette in a bottle (when it takes no more than a minute or two to whip up a fresh one that makes any salad fantastically delicious). That is American ingenuity and "convenience" at its worst.

I am such a stickler for proper nutrition that I don't want to send my kids to playdates with some of their junk food–loving classmates on weekends anymore—even though, of course, I do send them sometimes and I bite my tongue! But at home we bake together—my kids love to help me make my chocolate mousse or batches of cookies. Sweet treats are fine, of course, in moderation, and it's a wonderful time for my children and me when we spend happy hours making a mess in the kitchen and eating the results. They can learn good cooking and food-choice habits simply by watching what I'm preparing and helping me do it. And they're very happy with their snacks of fresh fruit, yogurt with jam or honey, or homemade smoothies with fruit, milk, and maple syrup.

If you need any more incentive—and want to lose weight, too—just watch *Fed Up,* a documentary by Katie Couric that the food industry doesn't want you to see. Or read the book *Salt Sugar Fat* by Michael Moss about the chemicals and preservatives food companies put in their most popular snacks to make sure you become addicted to their empty calories. And then start cooking!

SAVOR YOUR FOOD

We named our company Caudalie after the unit of measurement of wine left on your palate after you take a sip. The more caudalies, the more intense the flavor. Leave it to the French to come up with a poetic word for something so intangible—but it's what savoring your food is all about.

When we lived in Paris, my local *marché* in the Seventeenth Arrondissement was famous for its fresh fish like sole and bass, its gorgeous fruit and vegetables, and the truffle Camembert at the *fromagerie*. There was nothing more wonderful than strolling through the market in search of the freshest ingredients of the day. My local *poissonière* (fishmonger) knew that we liked sole; the baker handed me a *pain complet* (whole-grain bread); and La Dame de l'Auverge, the nickname we gave to the plum-cheeked fruit and veggies lady, always pointed to the peaches and homemade apricot jam that Bertrand especially loved.

The French *love* their food. We talk about meals and cooking the way Americans talk about sports. We know it's easy to savor what you eat when it is full of flavor. It's impossible to do when the food is full of chemicals, fake ingredients (ever read the label on your children's macaroni and cheese box? It's pretty scary!), high levels of sodium, and way too much sugar. When food is delicious, you want to inhale the divine aromas, chew it slowly, and enjoy every morsel. In fact, recent studies have shown that chewing and the enzymes saliva contains are deeply connected to proper digestion and maintaining a feeling of fullness after even small meals.

MODERATION, PLEASE!

Too much of anything, even the red wine I love, is never a good thing. When you're savoring your food, and when your food is savory, you will not want a lot of it. This can be hard to achieve in America, as our eyes (and stomachs) have adjusted to super-size portions, even if they're actually two or three times an intended serving. One easy way to shift this is to use smaller plates and utensils, clear them off the table when you're done, and not go back for seconds. Serve any leftovers the next day, so nothing goes to waste.

Not surprisingly, people tend to grossly underestimate the amount of calories they eat and drink during the day, and it's hard to fault them when they're served such enormous portions when they go out to eat. I was shocked when we arrived in America and a meal on my plate was enough for four people in France. I was even more shocked when I saw restaurants with salad bars or all-you-can-eat buffets. I know that an adult serving of protein is three to four ounces of steak, chicken, or fish—and that's only the size of your palm. A cup of cooked rice or pasta is only the size of your fist. When was the last time you saw that in a restaurant?

Plus, food labels can be very misleading. They break down the nutrients and calories, to be sure, but it's easy for your eyes to bypass the "Serving Size." You might think what you're eating is only one serving when it's actually three.

My thin and trim Parisian friends eat everything they want—they just eat small portions of it. They leave food on their plates if they aren't hungry. They don't ask for doggy bags, unless they have a doggy at home who likes leftover steak.

MEALTIMES ARE MEALTIMES

One day, not long ago, I was walking through our Bordeaux vineyard with someone from my American team, and she looked at her watch with a frown. "It's time for my protein," she told me as she pulled a PowerBar out of her purse. She ate it within seconds, and I realized that she'd just consumed what to her was lunch! I didn't have the heart to tell her that packaged protein bars aren't real food and they're loaded with sugar; it's a fallacy that they're really nutritious. She would have been much smarter to have eaten a crunchy green apple that would have given her phytonutrients and lots of fiber and taken more than a few seconds to eat and then had a nice, relaxed meal with me an hour or so later. By the time dinner rolled around, she was ravenous. And you know what that means.

One thing you will rarely see walking down a Parisian street is a Frenchwoman eating while they walk. I see this all day, every day, however, when I'm walking to my office in New York. People are eating and they don't even know what they're eating. If you're munching on the run, or standing up at your kitchen counters, or watching TV or streaming video or checking social media during meals, then mealtime becomes mindless eating time, and you won't have any idea how much you've actually consumed—or if you were even truly hungry for it.

The French sit down to eat. In the kitchen or the dining room. We see each mealtime as an important part of the day, as a time to enjoy each other's company, or, if we're alone, to enjoy our own company. No matter how fraught our workload, we stop and have a proper meal. It helps us calm our brains and bodies, and we know we will work more efficiently afterward.

It's very, very important to take that time to disconnect, no matter how busy you are. Don't eat at your desk. Find a space to sit down away from your computer and your phone and your devices. Even if it's just you, set the table, use a lovely plate and silverware, and relax. You need this time. You deserve it. It will help your digestion and it will help your mind and spirit, too!

EAT LIKE THE ROYALS

I like to joke with my children about how we eat like the royals:

- Eat breakfast like a king. Have it be the biggest, richest, and most satisfying meal of the day.

- Eat lunch like a prince. It's not quite as rich as breakfast, but still fills you up.

- Eat dinner like a peasant. This meal is just as delicious, but with nothing that takes a long time to digest.

In other words, breakfast should always be your biggest meal of the day and dinner your smallest. This gives your body the time it needs to efficiently process your meals. It keeps your blood sugar from spiking, which can give you uncontrollable cravings for carbohydrates and sugary snacks. And it gives you all the energy you need to make it through the day.

YOUR STOVE IS NOT THE ENEMY

It is a sad truth that the next generation of Frenchwomen is being raised on more fast food, but the majority of French people I know like to cook. I spent countless, happy hours in our *cuisine* when I was little, watching my grandmother whip up her delicious meals. She handed me a knife when I was only ten, and I was bursting with pride that she wanted (and expected) my help.

Because I grew up eating home-cooked meals every day, learning how to cook wasn't something that was difficult or a chore. I just knew what to do. So did my husband, who loves to make meals that are quick and satisfying, as I do. I have to admit that he's much better at making traditional dishes like osso buco à la Milanese than I am, so we tag-team our kitchen duty, as I prefer to cook veggies or seafood, make salads, and once in a while whip up my famous dark chocolate mousse.

I believe that cooking is one of those life skills that is truly essential. Not only do you control the amount of sugar, sodium, and fat in your food, but also your costs are far lower than if you bought packaged food or ate out. My children usually keep me company in the kitchen, and they see what I'm preparing, so the actual cooking process is demystified for them, as it was for me. It's a great time to talk about school and friends and everything else. We often spend a weekend afternoon in the kitchen, cooking our meals for the week that can then be stored in the freezer. If you don't have children, you can just as easily invite some friends over and cook some meals together. The time will fly by, and you'll not only have a lot of fun, but you'll also end up with healthy and nutritious meals that will encourage you to keep at it.

HOW I EAT ON A TYPICAL DAY

I eat a diet full of food that's energizing rather than energy-sapping—and it's just what my skin needs, too.

BREAKFAST

I eat breakfast every morning with my children. We have steel-cut oatmeal with fresh fruit and grilled *tartine* of good French bread with French butter and organic plum jam or raw honey. I have a cup of either Rooibos tea from Le Palais des Thés or Ladurée, or Kusmi Tea.

LUNCH

I like to have a large salad made with kale, quinoa, cranberries, goat cheese, Cajun chicken, grilled almonds, and cherry tomatoes, with a dressing of balsamic vinegar and olive oil. I also like sushi or fresh soup, depending on whether I am in the office or having a meeting over a meal.

SNACKS

As you know, I'm not much of a snacker. I keep organic apples, organic carrots, red grapes (preferably with seeds), other fruit, and almonds handy, and I have bowls of them out in the office for all my employees to eat. I also drink hot herbal tea loaded with antioxidants throughout the day. Caudalie organic herbal tea is very good for improving blood and lymph circulation (commonly referred to as "drainage") and is a delicious combination of red vine leaf, blackcurrant, blueberry, orange peel, and cinnamon.

DINNER

We love seafood. One of my favorite dishes to cook is fresh broiled scallops and quinoa or a salad of Burrata (fresh mozzarella), tomato, and fresh basil. I finish off both dishes with French sea salt (L'Île de Ré Sel de Guérande) and cold-pressed extra-virgin Italian olive oil. With a glass of red Château Smith Haut Lafitte, of course!

SUGAR IS A MORE LIKELY CULPRIT

Scientists have recently published numerous studies showing that fat might not be so bad for us after all. But sugar definitely is. American food is laden with the white stuff—often hidden in plain sight—and the American sweet tooth is definitely far stronger than the French one. That might be hard to believe if you're visiting Paris and walk by a *boulangerie* whose window is filled with almond croissants, all sorts of chocolate goodies, and enough pastries to fill Versailles. But those desserts are not eaten every day—they're special treats. We've never had the tradition of expecting a heavy, rich dessert after lunch or dinner—we're much more likely to order a cheese course that's served with some grapes or perhaps an apple. If you don't get in the habit of seeing something sweet as a reward, you don't care if you have it or not.

The epidemic of weight gain, metabolic syndrome (prediabetes), and type 2 diabetes is extremely dangerous for the health of children and adults. Dr. Kimber Stanhope, a nutritional biologist at the University of California, Davis, is a well-known expert investigating the effects of different sugars on metabolism, and her most recent study, "Adverse Metabolic Effects of Dietary Fructose: Results from the Recent Epidemiological, Clinical, and Mechanistic Studies," was published in 2013. Her studies, among others, show that eating simple carbohydrates (a piece of soft white sandwich bread, a bag of potato chips) or food high in sugar, particularly fructose (or high-fructose corn syrup) causes your pancreas to release large amounts of insulin, which then causes your blood sugar to spike as your body strives to find the correct balance. This sends the wrong signals to your brain, so that instead of metabolizing, or burning off, the sugar, it gets stored in your cells. And what is it stored as? You guessed it—*fat*. What's worse is that your brain then doesn't get the fuel it needs, so it sends off more signals telling your body it's hungry when it really isn't. This explains why drinking a glass of juice and eating a bagel or a donut for breakfast leaves you starving an hour or two later.

Knowing that, it does no one any harm and lots of people much good to have a Ladurée *macaron* once in a while. It's so delicious, and fills you up so quickly, and besides, you deserve a treat. A little bit of sugar is not the problem—eating it thoughtlessly and often is.

DON'T DRINK YOUR CALORIES

Do you know how many calories are in your extra-large latte with whipped cream? Or the fruit smoothie you think is good for you? As many as I ate for breakfast and lunch combined!

The problem with drinking calorie-dense beverages is that they're rarely filling, as they go down so quickly and easily, and it's very easy to underestimate the calorie count when you're thirsty. Frenchwomen are not in the habit of drinking as much juice or sodas as Americans, so it's easier for us to avoid them. We know they are overloaded with sugar and cause the insulin spikes that leave you even hungrier a short time later. For us, several glasses of mineral water or tea are more than enough.

Sugared drinks like soda have no nutritional value at all; they are made from high-fructose corn syrup and chemicals. In other words, they are the worst kind of junk. Fruit juice also has little nutritional value save for a bit of fiber and added vitamins, but it is still primarily sugar. And recent studies have shown that diet sodas can trigger insulin spikes, too, which could be one of the factors in weight gain for those who are trying hard to lose it. Artificially sweetened drinks often contain phosphorus, which can interfere with the absorption of calcium needed for strong bones. Ridding yourself of a soda habit is good for your body and your budget.

What I suggest is that you make a pot of tea in the morning and sip it all day. Sweeten it with a little raw honey if you need to, but try to taper that off. Many teas, like Rooibos, are full of nutrients and antioxidants and are also caffeine-free. Drinking them unsweetened gives you no calories and a lot of satisfaction.

DON'T SNACK YOUR CALORIES, EITHER

When French children come home from school, they usually expect to have a little *goûter*—a snack (it translates to "a taste"). This might be some raw almonds or a piece of fruit—nothing more. It fills them up, gives them energy for homework or playtime, yet doesn't spoil their appetite for a nutritious dinner. Because we tend not to snack, we are hungry for good food at mealtimes. If you haven't eaten any junk all day, it's pretty amazing what you *can* eat at your meals, particularly vegetables, salads, and whole grains that are loaded with fiber that quickly fill you up.

If you find yourself hungry between meals, don't starve yourself. Eat something nutritious and filling. Just try not to snack after dinner, as that can affect your digestion, keeping you awake.

EATING WELL ISN'T JUST GOOD FOR YOUR SKIN (THE FRENCH PARADOX)

In America, heart disease causes nearly two-thirds of deaths annually—thanks to risk factors such as obesity, diabetes and other weight-related illnesses, smoking, overconsumption of alcohol, and stress. A diet laden with artery-clogging saturated fat, which is found in meat and dairy products, is one of the primary culprits.

So why don't the French, who love their Camembert and fresh butter and rare roast beef, have the same high levels of heart disease? Despite clinical factors that are comparable to those in other countries (high blood pressure, lots of smoking, not enough exercise), a much lower rate of French people die from heart attacks; statistics show that there are approximately 36 to 55 percent fewer in France than in America.

In 1980, scientists launched a study of seven thousand people to explore the perplexing phenomenon that had been dubbed the French paradox, and other studies have since confirmed the original findings. Scientists found that the more you eat vegetables, fruits, and vegetable oils (like olive)—what's become known as the Mediterranean diet—the lower your risk for coronary disease. Do you think that this diet rich in antioxidants and EFAs that are so good for your skin might have something to do with that? I certainly do.

Yet even if the Mediterranean diet is partly responsible for this paradox, it does not explain why the French have a significantly lower heart attack rate than its neighboring Mediterranean countries such as Spain or Italy. (The only other industrialized country that has a better score is Japan.) Although the French eat more fresh vegetables than the English or the Americans, the average diet is also often full of foie gras, full-fat cheeses, sausages, and the occasional croissant, all of which contain enormous amounts of saturated fats. The French consumption of saturated fat is, in fact, very similar to countries with a high death rate due to coronary disease, such as Scotland, and the cholesterol rate is similar to many other countries, too.

The *only* thing that distinguishes France from other countries is its wine-drinking habits. On average, a French adult drinks about one hundred bottles of wine each year. (Italy comes in second, with an average of eighty-seven bottles.) And, coincidently, the lowest level of heart attacks is found in the south of France, particularly in Toulouse, with seventy-eight deaths due to heart attacks per one hundred thousand citizens. This isn't due to the gorgeous, sun-drenched weather or the splendor of the countryside—it's because the southern French eat more fruits and vegetables and drink more red wine.

In 1991, a physician named Serge Renaud discussed this paradox in the French media, and his conclusions were eventually shared on a celebrated segment of the CBS-TV show *60 Minutes* (the same one that Professor Vercauteren had discussed with us the day he visited the vineyard). "Red wine is one of the strongest remedies in order to decrease death rates related to coronary diseases," Dr. Renaud stated. Needless to say, wine sales skyrocketed all over America after that pronouncement.

As you'll learn in part 2, the high resveratrol content of red wine is what provides so many health benefits. That's what makes a moderate amount of wine so good for you. As well as so delicious!

HOW TO DRINK RED WINE
LIKE THE FRENCH

The ideal temperature to serve red wine is about 65 degrees. Try, if you can, to store red wine at about 55 degrees. Your basement can often do quite well, or you can use a small wine refrigerator if you become serious about different wines.

- Open the wine bottle at least one hour before you plan to drink it, to give it time to breathe. This will deepen its flavor.

- Always hold the glass by its stem. This lets you judge its color, and not warm it up.

- Use all your senses to taste. Many professional wine tasters look at the color of the wine before they drink but then close their eyes when they're sipping so they can focus on the caudalies, scent, and feel.

- Start with the first nose. Try to name all the many flavors you can distinguish simply by inhaling the initial aroma.

- The second nose is when you oxygenate the wine in the glass. The aromas blossom and become more concentrated. Try to name them now and see what's different.

- Take a sip of wine and swirl it around until it covers your entire palate. It's okay to "chew" on it.

- Count the wine caudalies once you've swallowed the wine; each one is approximately one second. (Think of them as the aftertaste that remains on your palate.) The more there are, the better the wine. What I love about caudalies is that they're unique. They're not a science—just as no perfume smells exactly the same on different wearers, so wine tasters sipping the same wine will experience different caudalies.

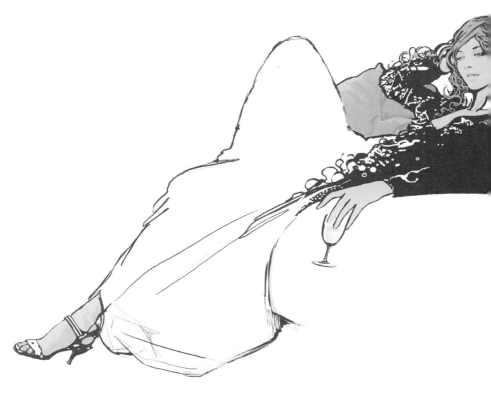

Three

RELAXATION À LA FRANÇAISE

The best beauty secret I ever learned came to me from my great-grandmother: Drink one glass of red wine every day, and have at least one thirty-minute walk. She died at the age of 103 after a hardworking life in the mountains of France, so *voilà!*

I knew all about those mountains. When, like so many teenagers, I wanted a bit of escape from our farm, I would hop on my bicycle and ride the narrow roads that wound their way up and down the mountain. Or I'd go for hikes on weekends with my friends, and we'd start in our backyard, where my father built several small waterfalls in the stream that meandered through our property, filling our ears with its soothing sound as we looked for tadpoles. These outdoor adventures always brought roses to my cheeks and left me strong and fit even when I wasn't even thinking about the need for exercise. My friends and I were just always on the go.

I may have dreamed of escaping to the city when I was

younger, but once I did move to Paris and then to New York, I had to find ways to recharge myself as I was once able to do with such ease in the countryside. I went from breathing in crisp, clean mountain air to inhaling vast amounts of pollution and cigarette smoke; from nights whose noises came only from the crickets and the owls to endless sirens and traffic and chatter.

Life is complicated. Nearly all the women I know, French or American, struggle with the constant pull on our energy to manage everything we need to do—days filled with work, childcare, household management, and trying to find some time for ourselves, our friends, and our partners. Trying to juggle all the balls I have up in the air at one time can leave me flat instead of flying. How do I find that balance? How can *you* balance all the demands confronting you? And, since this is a book about beauty, how do I manage it all without compromising my style or routines? There's a fundamental flaw in thinking all these things are mutually exclusive—that you can either be busy and successful or relaxed and happy. In reality, in order to be as successful as you can be, you can't forget to take care of yourself. There may be a million things to do on any given day, but I never let self-care take a backseat to any of it. It may be the most important thing on my calendar.

MANAGING YOUR STRESS

Stress shows on your face.

It doesn't matter how beautiful you are or may have been. If you've lived a fulfilling existence, both professionally and personally, and if you've had good, solid relationships, the results are visible. If life has been hard, or if you've recently faced challenging situations (such as problems at work) or emotionally devastating situations (such as the death of loved ones, or divorce, or moving), that will show as well. It's not a myth that hair can go white overnight due to extreme emotional trauma—many cases have been documented throughout history.

Stress management is a crucial part of any beauty routine. When we're stressed, our bodies produce a jolt of adrenaline and other hormones called glucocorticoids. These chemicals were particularly useful thousands of years ago when humans needed all their wits about them just to survive another day. Now, we no longer live with this danger, but our bodies still respond to stress with floods of these chemicals. The long-term result is visible in the skin.

Doubtless you already know what stressed skin looks like: Its natural color is off, either ashen or yellow tinged. Cheeks may be flushed. Think of college students pulling all-nighters to cram for exams; they look blotchy, bloated, and sallow. And those circles under your eyes—well, never mind those! Even your favorite cucumber compresses can't make a dent in them.

In addition, stress can make lines and wrinkles seem more pronounced. Breakouts can sprout, especially around the jawline, even in those who haven't had acne for years. Skin can be unusually dry, with scaly patches. Cheeks can droop and chins can sag. Hair looks limp and blah and can even start to fall out. Autoimmune skin diseases such as eczema and psoriasis can reappear. Wounds take longer to heal and it takes longer for our bodies to fight off disease.

Stress has become such a frequent companion to our days that we don't even realize just how overwhelmed we actually are. The solution is to try to keep on as even a keel as possible.

And while the French can certainly be masters of snobbery, I think our attitude toward life is much more *laissez-faire* than what I've seen in New York, where competitiveness overshadows what you'd think would be the simplest things. For example, when I wanted to put my children in a dance class, I was appalled to find they had to audition first! The children who did get into this class had to hire private coaches to teach them what to do before they were accepted. Can you imagine? I feel for these children, as they have the kind of type-A tiger moms who need to excel (and have their children excel) or their world falls apart. That is too much pressure on anyone, especially a child. My mother had high standards for my behavior and my academic work, but other than that she insisted on only one thing: that I had to be able to be comfortable with any kind of people. It was just as important for me to treat the baker's son and the butcher's daughter with the same regard as I would treat the children of a wealthy socialite. That has served me very well and I've tried to instill the same values in my kids and protect them from the unnecessary stress of having to excel at everything.

Get Enough Sleep

Do you get enough sleep? I try to, but it can be very difficult when I'm on the road, have jet lag, and need to be up and bright-eyed for presentations or to do meet-and-greets in locations all over the world. And it can be just as difficult when I'm in New York and life is just too busy!

Being tired makes you hungry, nervous, and grumpy. (At least that's how I feel!) According to the National Sleep Foundation, lack of sleep doesn't just give you dark circles under your eyes or make them puffy. It can be very dangerous for your health, leading to an increased risk of heart problems, diabetes, psychiatric conditions, stroke, other chronic conditions, and weight gain—to say nothing of the risks of drowsy driving and a decreased ability to pay attention and be at your best.

In addition, chronic sleep problems can wreak visible havoc

on your skin, as the stress hormones that get released can break down collagen, which is what gives your skin its elasticity. Deep sleep is also the time when human growth hormone is released, and you need it to keep your bones, muscles, and skin strong.

The National Institutes of Health has stated that fifty to seventy million Americans are affected by a lack of sleep. That's near epidemic levels. You can use any of the relaxation tips in the next section to prepare your body for sleep, but if your day is still too crammed and the alarm needs to go off too early, you will still feel the effects of sleep deprivation.

When I'm exhausted, I spritz the scent of Caudalie's Crème Tisane de Nuit, made with basil, chamomile, lemongrass, lavender, mint, orange blossom, and thyme, around my pillow. The aroma therapeutic scents sooth my mind and soul and help relax me. I recently began using the 4/7/8 method a friend told me about: Simply inhale for four seconds through your nose, hold your breath for seven seconds, then exhale for eight seconds through your mouth until you fall asleep. This kind of focused breathing is an excellent way to relax, as concentrating on your breath in such an unusual way helps clear your mind of all those nagging thoughts and worries that can keep you awake. It's actually a form of meditation, and if you practice it enough, you'll be able to use it to relieve stress whenever you need to.

RELAXATION FOR BEAUTIFUL SKIN

Rapid, shallow breathing is synonymous with stress. It may also release damaging free radicals. Breathing consciously and slowly relieves stress instantly. It sounds silly, but it's true. Inhale to the count of three, then slowly exhale to the count of three. Deep breathing also stops you from yelling at your kids when they've opened a bag of flour in the kitchen and decided to play with it . . . all over the house! Yoga, Pilates, and meditation classes can help tremendously with teaching people how to breathe effectively. Try to find at least a few minutes each day where you do nothing more complicated than focusing on your breathing—this is also the essence of meditation, another known stress-buster.

When Frenchwomen need to catch their breath and decompress, they head for a day spa. Just as there are nail salons on practically every corner of Manhattan's streets, it seems to be the same for *instituts de beauté* in Paris. Because they're so ubiquitous and inexpensive, it's not uncommon for us to get a facial at least once or twice a month. One of my favorite estheticians, a lovely lady named Régine who now works at the Caudalie Spa at the Plaza Hotel in New York City, does an amazingly rejuvenating facial. She gently pinches your skin with her fingertips—what we call *pincement de jaquet* (a face massage without use of a cream or oil, consisting of tiny pinches between the thumb and the index finger to firm and tone as well as stimulate the skin) and *palpe roule* (a rolling massage), which is a marvel at improving your lymphatic drainage and smoothing out your skin. It may sound a bit odd but it's incredibly soothing and has the added bonus of giving you a mini-lift that lasts for several days.

Regular facials not only have wonderful effects on your stress levels, but they also have a noticeable effect on your skin. You can have one, as Régine says, no matter what shape your skin is in. Even those with acne are terrific candidates, as a good beauty therapist will ensure that your oil glands are balanced and your skin gets the hydration it needs to reduce further oil production that can cause breakouts.

This is a perfect example of the Pleasure Principle. We know that a little bit of pampering isn't just a luxury—it's a necessity to help you de-stress and take you away from the constant pressures of modern life. Plus, there seems to be a cumulative effect, so the more you go, the more results you'll see on your skin.

Frenchwomen don't give a second thought to telling their friends, family, or colleagues, "I need some time for myself." We just do it. Even if you don't think you deserve a break (and you do!), an hour or two in a spa is an ideal way to show you not only how to relax, but also that you've earned every peaceful and soothing second you'll spend in there.

Furthermore, you don't need a lot of money or a spare week to go to a spa for your ultimate fantasy vacation in order to reap the benefits. One full day is like giving you a week off; a half day is like giving you a weekend of bliss; and a quick facial at lunchtime will recharge your day. Even better, you can talk to your estheticians and get some wonderful ideas about incorporating as many spa techniques as possible into your daily life.

French Beauty Secret

One of the French stress-busters we all love is sex. Not only is it one of the great joys of life, but time with your lover actually improves your circulation and brings the most delicious roses to your cheeks. It gives you that certain glow, *bien sur!* No wonder Nars named his bestselling blush "Orgasm"!

Follow the advice of one of my friends' Parisian grandmother: "Always coordinate your lingerie," she says. "Because you never know what might happen."

Spending the time you need and deserve on making yourself feel better is hardly a waste of time—it is actually an extremely *efficient* use of your time. When you're refreshed, relaxed, or energized, it's so much easier to tackle everything else on your to-do list, more efficiently and with greater ease.

CREATING A RELAXING SPA ATMOSPHERE AT HOME

Whenever you walk into any of the Caudalie spas, your senses are immediately engaged—and the mood is set. If you've ever been to one of these spas or any other one, you know that's a deliberate part of the overall experience. The air will be perfumed with a relaxing scent, and there will be soft music playing, or perhaps a fountain with the soothing sound of rushing water. Voices will be low. The lights will be dim, with candles flickering, and the chairs are always extra-comfortable. You'll change into a bathrobe that will be thick and plush, and your cell phone will be turned off. You will be handed a cup of herbal tea or a glass of lemon-infused water. Within a few minutes, you've already started to unwind.

Fortunately, you don't have to spend a lot of money, or even leave the house, to get this same experience. You can easily create your own mini-spa at home with these super-simple and inexpensive tips that engage all your senses.

Scent: The easiest way to create a relaxing spa atmosphere at home is by stimulating the most potent of your senses. It's all about scent. Burning a delectably fragranced candle is the quickest way to transport you out of the everyday. This has been proven by more than thirty years of studies undertaken by International Flavors & Fragrances, Inc. (IFF), one of the largest suppliers of raw fragrances to perfumers in the world.

Find a scent or scents that evoke strong memories of something pleasurable or wonderful in your life. It could be a vanilla that reminds you of your grandmother's sugar cookies. Or lavender—for that trip you took to the south of France where you wandered through acres of ripening plants waving gently in the wind. Or sandalwood—for the time you went to Chinatown in San Francisco and got caught in the rain only to discover that the little sandalwood fan you'd just bought smelled even more delicious when it was wet. I love lighting candles that smell like the vine flower—yes, it grows on grapevines!—because the scent reminds me of our vineyard in Bordeaux at the end of spring, when you can feel that summer is soon to arrive.

You can also use aromatherapy to perfume your environment. You'll learn more about this in chapter 5, but essential oils are highly concentrated essences of different herbs and flowers, and they all have different properties. At the Caudalie spas, we create concentrated aromatherapy blends containing high percentages of different organic essential oils such as juniper berry, rosemary, and geranium for toning, and organic essential oils of lemongrass and lemon for lymphatic drainage. Add a few drops of your favorite essential oil in the corner of a shower stall or bath and let the hot running water carry the scent into the air as you relax in the water. Or you can get a diffuser that will gently heat the oil, allowing it to flood your room with scent.

Do be careful with these oils, however, as they are extremely concentrated, so you should never apply them full-strength to your skin; a few drops are all you need to stir into a cream or to add to bathwater. I like to use bergamot, neroli (orange blossom), and petitgrain (lemon leaf) oil in a warm bath as an instant de-stressor. I also enjoy dabbing mint oil–infused cream on the nape of my neck to wake me up in the morning and sprinkling lavender oil onto my pillow just before bedtime to help me sleep.

I'll show you how to use essential oils to customize your skincare products in chapter 5. Fill your bathroom with your favorite scents, and you'll always have a lovely smelling sanctuary to which you can retreat whenever you're feeling stressed or run-down or just need a few private moments to revitalize yourself.

Touch: If you prefer showers to baths, use a scented shower gel lathered onto damp skin. Afterward, apply a rich and hydrating body cream while your skin is still damp to help lock in extra moisture. Don't forget your feet! Slather on a revitalizing foot cream to relieve tired soles. Put on a pair of cotton socks to help the cream soak in and prevent you from sliding around. This will also help the cream be absorbed with maximum potency.

French Beauty Secret

Try finishing your bath or shower with cold water
for an energy boost and immediate firming effect.

Taste: Depending on the time of day, make yourself a warm cup of fragrant herbal tea or pour yourself a glass of red wine. Sip it while you're in the bath or winding down elsewhere.

When I want to relax, I choose an organic tea made with either catnip, melissa, valerian, verbena, linden, passionflower, motherwort, or blue vervain, as they are all calming and soothing. The one that works best for me is valerian, even if it tastes a bit peculiar. Valerian is well-known as a sleep aid and helps reduce tension. (A funny aside—valerian root contains a chemical called valeranone, which is similar to nepetalactone, the active chemical in catnip. My Parisian cat Popcorn loved it any time I had valerian tea!)

Sight: Dimming the lights while you bathe or shower helps calm and sooth you. Try lighting candles instead of turning on the electric lights. If you bathe at night, the darkness will help prepare you for sleep. If you shower during the day and have a window in your bathroom, let the natural light fill the space.

You can also use color to enhance a relaxing mood, as different colors have different effects on your mood—something hospital administrators have discovered, as bright colors improve the well-being of their patients. According to Colour Affects, a professional trade organization in the United Kingdom that has extensively studied how colors affect people, the most soothing colors are pink, blue, green, yellow, and lilac. But, of course, any color that you find particularly enticing and relaxing will do the trick. You don't have to settle for a boring white bathroom; it's really amazing how a few coats of paint can utterly transform a room and a mood.

Sound: Turn on any kind of music that is soothing and transports you. Make sure the beat is slow and steady and the music isn't too loud or jangly or you'll find it hard to relax. You can do this in the morning, too, when you're getting ready for the day. Music that's upbeat and that makes you feel happy will automatically put you in a good mood—and what better way to face all your tasks than in a relaxed state of mind?

HOW TO GIVE YOURSELF A FACIAL AT HOME

Facials done by a trained esthetician who understands your skin are an absolute marvel and a regular part of my skincare routine. Doing a facial at home can't give you quite the same experience but will still leave you feeling refreshed, cleansed, and hydrated. Here are my favorite tips from Régine Berthelot, Caudalie's master facialist:

- Use a gentle cleanser to clean your face; follow up with a hydrating toner; exfoliate lightly if you need it; open up your pores with a bit of steam to release any toxins; tone one more time to make sure your pores are clean; massage in a serum or oil; then finish with a mask of your choice, depending on your skin's needs.

- Don't be overzealous with your cleansing. Gentle cleansing does the trick without stripping your skin of natural oils. Alternate or combine different cleansers depending on different needs. If you were outside on a blustery day, for example, your skin might be drier and more chapped than usual. In that case, mix a cleansing milk with a cleansing oil for extra creaminess. Rinse with water. A foam cleanser or soap is usually better for oilier skin. Follow that with a hydrating toner, preferably one that is gentle and alcohol-free. It's important to use a gentle toner that won't strip your skin of oil because doing so causes your oil glands to overcompensate by creating more oil in an effort to lubricate what they're perceiving as overly dry skin. This is why anyone with acne or troubled skin can still have a facial—proper hydration *reduces* the amount of oil your skin produces.

- Gently exfoliate after you cleanse and tone, but no more than once or twice a week. All you want to do is slough off the dead skin cells, so avoid any harsh scrubs that contain ground-up apricot pits or any large pieces of an abrasive material that can tear pores and do more harm than good. Regular proper exfoliation can "teach" your skin to react the right way; if you faithfully exfoliate every seven days, your skin will come to expect this and won't overreact during the other six days.

- Professional estheticians often use a steaming machine to add moisture to the air and to your skin, and the wet heat gradually opens your pores and rids your skin of impurities. It's hard to mimic this at home, but the best way is by turning on the shower and leaving the door or curtain open so the steam fills the room, using a hot steam vaporizer or humidifier in a small room, or placing your face over a bowl of extremely hot water (draping a towel around your head if you like) for a few minutes.

- Massage your face to improve circulation and lymphatic drainage. Your lymphatic system removes waste from your body, so stimulating it helps the process and minimizes water retention—that's why the word *drainage* is used—which is what causes bloating and puffiness. When you apply your cleanser, massage it in with big round circular motions. Use your entire hand, not just your fingertips. Do it in a rhythmical beat—use your heartbeat as a guide—and that will be wonderfully relaxing.

- Be sure to massage in a therapeutic serum or oil after your face is cleansed. Pressing on pressure points for your facial nerves is also a great stress-buster. One of the best areas to press is your "third eye"—the area right between your eyebrows. This is the center of all the nerve endings in your face, which is why, when you're stressed, you tend to break out in that area. (Important point: Never squeeze any pimples there, as this can swell up your eyes.) Other pressure points are found on your temples, and all around the orbital bones of your eyes, so press on them from above your eyes to underneath them. This will help get rid of dark circles and puffiness and help relieve any congestion. Lastly, press above and underneath your lips.

- To enhance lymphatic drainage, start in the center of your forehead and use broad strokes downward with your fingertips, smoothing the skin from the center to the side. Next, stroke around your eyes, then around your chin and jaw. Always use these draining movements from the top down as your biggest lymph nodes for your upper body are located in your underarms, and you want to move the lymphatic fluid toward them.

- Next, apply the mask of your choice. While the mask is working, try massaging your hands, arms, and feet to help you relax even more—or better yet see if someone else (perhaps your lover?) will do this for you. Or try doing your facials with a friend, as you can massage each other's faces and feel even

French Beauty Secret

The Herboristerie du Palais Royal is a hidden gem in the First Arrondissement of Paris where everyone I know goes to get their specially blended essential oils. It's a stunning experience just walking into the apothecary, because it's so old and it smells so wonderful and it's a treat for all your senses. They used to make up an elixir for me, containing rosemary, mint, melissa, orange blossom, myrrh, rose, and benzoin, following the centuries-old recipe of Queen Isabelle of Hungary. It always made my skin feel and smell delicious.

better. If you're very tired, you can skip this step. Lie down with your mask on and relax. You can put anything cold, like tea bags or a cool washcloth, on your eyes to reduce puffiness.

• Remove your mask with lukewarm water and a soft washcloth and apply a serum and moisturizer. You should definitely have the glow!

HOW THE FRENCH EXERCISE

They don't!

Or rather, compared to the highly driven women I see in New York City, they certainly don't organize their days around their workouts. I was astonished when I moved to New York and saw women jogging on city blocks or in Central Park, pushing their babies or toddlers in strollers, when the sun was just starting to rise. I looked at them with awe and admiration—but trust me, no Parisian mom would *ever* do such a thing, even if she needed the exercise. We are much too lazy.

I wish I could tell you there was some special form of French exercise that helps keep us slim. There isn't. We don't exercise nearly as much as Americans do. We don't particularly like gyms or energetic classes that leave you drenched in sweat. In fact, even though there are more joggers in the Luxembourg Gardens now than there were a decade ago (but not in the wee hours, which is when Central Park is teeming with exercisers), I've yet to meet a Parisienne who thought running there was the best way to get in shape. That's a shame. We are very aware of the cardiovascular benefits of regular exercise; we all want flat abs and toned thighs. We all know that it brings a healthy glow to skin and helps us maintain a healthy weight. It's a great way to zone out and decompress, too. We just don't like to do the hard work.

That said, I am rather unusual for a Frenchwoman, as my parents were top athletes—they met and fell in love on the ski slopes in Val d'Isère and my dad was on the French Olympic team in the 1960s. They are both still incredibly active and spend as much time on skis as they can in winter months.

My mother, in fact, still has a ridiculous amount of energy. Her job running the vineyard with my father keeps her on her feet, and she also hikes a lot or bikes around the property in the summer and skis as much as possible in the winter. Once a week she does Pilates along with an on-demand exercise show on TV. And she has absolutely not one dimple of cellulite, much to the envy of my much-younger friends.

I also love to ski in the winter and do all kinds of water sports in the summer, but organized sports and workouts in the gym have never been my style. I prefer to bike to work, or walk when I have the time. It clears my head for the day ahead and doesn't take too much time away from my busy schedule.

Even Frenchwomen who roll their eyes at the American tourists in their exercise sneakers—something they would never, ever wear out in public, unless they were designed by Prada or Comme des Garçons!—secretly envy the ease with which American women incorporate their workouts into their daily routine, effortlessly going from the office to the gym to a dinner or evening out with friends. What we do instead is small increments of exercise— and yes, these are very beneficial. It takes very little time for muscles to respond to being used, and every minute counts. A little bit of exercise is a lot better than none.

So instead of long runs, Frenchwomen love brisk walks. Paris is such a lovely city, and there are so many wonderful things to see, that it's easy to have those regular strolls even if the point is not to exercise but to seek out a new *marché* or used bookstore. If you live in an area that's not conducive to daily walking—suburban America, for example, or a city like Los Angeles where a car is a must—park your car farther away from your office building or the shopping center, use the stairs whenever possible, and try to schedule walks during lunchtime or breaks at work. Lots of my French friends have dogs, which means they're out walking them several times a day, too.

We also have a weekly yoga hour for all Caudalie employees in New York and Paris. It's a terrific way to decompress, concentrate on breathing, get stronger, and be encouraged to keep at it.

THE FRENCH LOVE THEIR *VACANCES*

When the French go on strike, it's serious business. The entire country practically shuts down until terms are negotiated, and one of the most beloved and nonnegotiable of the French workers' expectations is a lot of time off. For us, the month of August is the sacred month of shutdown where practically everyone goes on vacation (except the people in the service industry, who are happy for the business). We have several weeks at the end of December, and French law mandates that employees are given five (yes, *five!*) weeks of paid vacation, and women are given at least sixteen weeks (for the first and second child) to twenty-six weeks (for the third child) and thirty-four weeks for twins of paid maternity leave.

The French have a much different attitude toward time off—we know that stressed, exhausted, and frustrated workers are not efficient. We know bodies need a break from the daily grind of getting to and from work, even if you love your job. I must say, though, that the American tendency to have national holidays on Mondays, giving you long weekends, is much smarter than what the French do. Our national holidays, which happen pretty much every month, fall in the middle of the week, which disrupts everyone's work schedules. It's inefficient, but it's certainly in character.

When my family goes on vacation, we generally just head to the countryside to chill. Americans often find it hard to relax and do nothing. They are so used to being busy that their vacation time is planned to the nanosecond with activities. I understand that, especially if you don't have a lot of vacation time and want to make the most of it, or if you've traveled a long way and want to take advantage of your new surroundings. But I still believe the best vacation to de-stress is the vacation where you do nothing. Or rather, you do nothing more intense than go to the pool or for a walk in the morning, have a siesta in the afternoon, and a long, lingering dinner in the twilight. In France, we will plan—if that's the word!—lots of these dinners. We'll go to the local *marché* in the morning and buy whatever suits our fancy; we'll cook a simple meal; and we'll invite our friends over to share the meal. Someone will open a bottle of an *aperitif* and we'll have cocktails before sitting down to eat. For me, this is the purest essence of happiness and relaxation: good food, good wine, good friends, and good company. That is the perfect vacation for me. I know how recharged I am afterward. My skin is glowing and my brain is working a mile a minute because I gave it a break and calmed down all those busy work-related thoughts. A do-nothing vacation always sparks my creativity—so while I might do nothing during the trip, I certainly do a lot more afterward!

We believe that life is a marathon, not a sprint, so you learn to pace yourself accordingly. If I were an American, I am pretty sure when I was starting my company I would have worked through every summer and never taken the sick days allotted to me like so many of my American friends. As a result, I likely would have been completely burned out and too miserable to work effectively or with any passion and might have ended up having to sell my business because I couldn't keep up. Instead, by knowing how much time I have off, and what relaxing plans I'll have in August with my family, I give my brain and body the time I know I need to disconnect. It makes me a much happier and healthier worker the rest of the year.

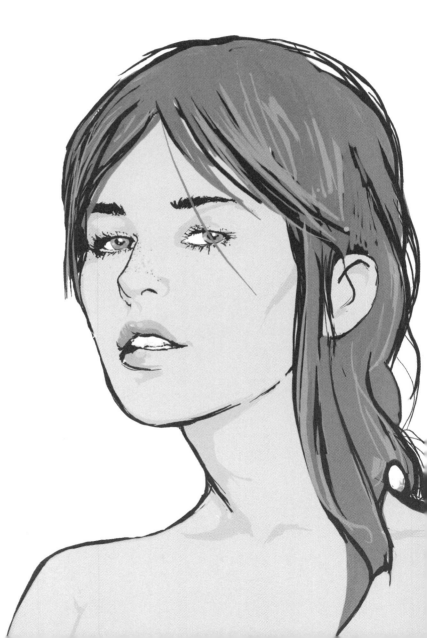

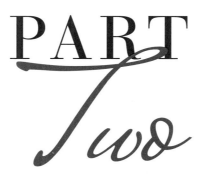

PART
Two

Skin Basics

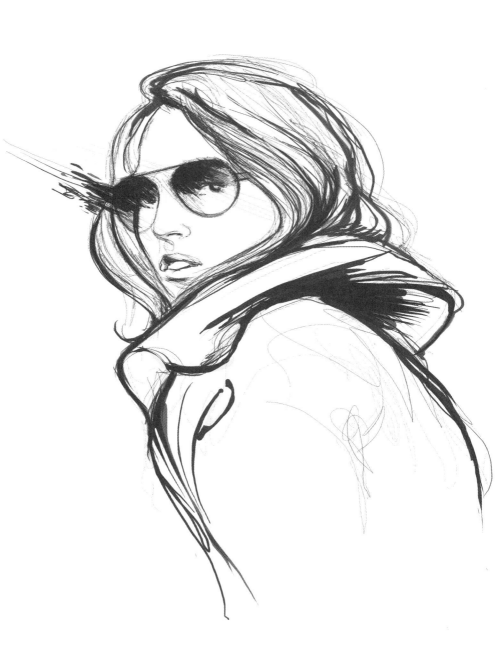

Four

HOW YOUR SKIN AGES

When we think of "organs," we either think about that imposing musical instrument in Notre-Dame Cathedral, or maybe your kidneys or liver. We rarely think of our skin even though it's our body's largest organ, covering twenty square feet and making up 15 percent of your total weight. Obviously, it's also the only organ that is constantly exposed to the elements. Even when bombarded by sun and wind, hot and cold, it's a marvel of constant replenishment, and if you understand exactly how it works, you will be better prepared to protect and repair it no matter your age or lifestyle.

Skin is made up of three layers:

- Epidermis—top layer

  The top, living layer of the skin is the epidermis. Approximately 80 to 95 percent of it is composed of short-lived keratinocytes that have migrated up to the surface. When they do, they die and are transformed into corneocytes, forming a topmost layer called the stratum corneum. This layer forms a protective shield preventing bacteria, excess water, and other elements from entering your body, and it also prevents the loss of water and minerals. The epidermis also contains melanocytes, which produce the melanin that gives your skin its color and may form spots; as well Langerhans cells, which are your skin's first defense against germs, sending white blood cells to fight off any viruses or bacteria when you get a cut or scrape.

- Dermis—middle layer

  The middle layer of skin is the dermis, or dermal layer. Up to 70 percent of the dermis is composed of collagen, an interconnective tissue made from protein that provides structure, firmness, and elasticity. The dermis also contains elastin, another protein fiber that's responsible for your skin's elasticity, as well as nerves, blood vessels, sweat glands, the hair follicles for your body hair, and sebaceous (oil) glands, GAG (glycoaminoglycanes), and fibroblasts.

- Subcutaneous or hypodermis—bottom layer

  The subcutaneous skin layer is made of fat cells called adipocytes. These cells store energy and contribute to your skin's volume—it's the kind of good fat that gives babies such irresistible dumpling cheeks that you just want to pinch. Without this fat, you'd have no insulation or protection for your internal organs. In addition, some sweat glands, sebaceous glands, and the follicles for the hair on your head are located here.

WHAT AGES OUR SKIN

There are two types of factors that age your skin: intrinsic (the natural aging process you can't really control) and extrinsic (factors you have more control over).

INTRINSIC AGING

Dermatologists often joke that skin starts to age as soon as we're born, but the signs of aging don't typically start for women until we're in our mid to late twenties. At first there will be tiny wear-and-tear lines, depending on your skin habits, and they usually go away. By the time you're in your late twenties and beyond, though, these tiny lines tend to stick around as your skin loses resilience. That's because, as you get older, all your cell functions start to slow down, everywhere in your body. When cells don't replenish as well as they once did, your face is less able to repair damage, your muscles and bones become weaker, and your energy levels decrease.

Intrinsic aging is modulated by your genetic predisposition, your DNA, hormone levels, illnesses, and/or poor nutrition, which can stress and damage skin. And let's not forget gravity, which pulls down and elongates noses and earlobes and feet over the years (what a charming thought!). Intrinsic aging is also responsible for the following:

- The epidermis becomes thicker and the junction between the epidermis and the dermis becomes flatter, which makes it harder for your skin to bounce back.

- Expression lines, or wrinkles, appear as a result of constant use of your facial muscles. A wrinkle is a line, furrow, or crease on your skin—it's actually a scar triggered by an inflammatory response to damage in the deeper skin layers.

Wrinkles appear due to repetitive motion, particularly around your eyes and mouth, along your nose, and on your forehead.

- Collagen production decreases and elastin fibers begin to sag and break, so skin is less resilient. At the same time, the fat levels decrease and the facial bones can shrink slightly (which is a natural part of the aging process), which is why those with a low percentage of body fat can look a lot older than they are. This loss of dimensionality, or volume, is a huge factor in aging.

- Your hair follicles are rooted in your sebaceous glands, and pores are the passageways from these glands up to the skin's surface. As we age, there's a double whammy of sebaceous glands growing larger coupled with a slower turnover of skin cells within each pore. (Fortunately, it's easy to treat pores with peeling/exfoliating products containing glycolic acid or papaya enzymes, as they work really well. Just don't overdo any scrubbing, because that will only further irritate the edges of your pores and make things worse! See the section on page 128 in chapter 5 for more.)

- Melanocyte production decreases, so there is less pigment in the skin.

- Langerhans cells, which work with your immune system to help fight infections, decrease in number. You'll bruise more easily and take longer to heal.

- The sebaceous glands produce less oil, so skin becomes drier.

- Hair follicles decrease in number.

You have no more control over your own body's intrinsic aging than you do over the texture of your hair or the color of your eyes.

(Sagging, for example, is due as much to intrinsic aging, depending on your fat stores and the effect of gravity on them, as it is to extrinsic aging, especially if you have a lot of sun damage.) Take a look at your mother and get used to what you see because you tend to age as your parents do.

Not all skin ages the same way: People of color, especially those with dark skin, tend to age better, as the larger amount of pigment in their skin helps give them more protection from the sun. Some ethnicities, especially those of Asian descent, tend to have more rounded faces, with a thicker layer of fat in the subcutaneous layer. The more fat there is, the more volume and the more youthful you will appear. Men also don't age as quickly as women, as they have a thicker dermis, with deeper and more numerous hair follicles. This helps support the skin structure—and their regular shaving naturally exfoliates all those dead skin cells on the epidermis.

Fortunately, intrinsic aging is responsible for only about 20 percent of the skin's signs of aging before the ages of fifty-five to sixty. And the work of anti-aging scientists, including Dr. David Sinclair at the Harvard Medical School, may someday be able to alter how cells age. I'll discuss this more in chapter 5.

EXTRINSIC AGING

The other 80 percent or so of signs of premature skin aging (such as wrinkles and pigmentation disorders), is due to extrinsic, or outside, sources that you often can control:

- Sun exposure from UV (ultraviolet) radiation (see the section starting on page 100 in this chapter). What most people think of as aging—brown spots, enlarged pores, uneven skin tone, wrinkles, spots, or a dull, lifeless complexion—is actually due primarily to photoaging, or damage from the sun's powerful radiation. Compare the skin on your face to the skin on your belly, which is rarely exposed to sunshine, and you can instantly see the difference.

- Smoking. See the sidebar on page 95 for the gory details!

- Environmental stresses. If the air is very dirty where you live, it's not only attacking your skin from the outside, but also forcing you to inhale noxious particles that cause harm from the inside out. Climate, particularly air that is very dry or very cold, also adversely affects skin.

- Stress levels. Your loved ones always know when you're not getting enough sleep or are weighed down by too much stress because it shows in your skin. Many studies have shown how stress ages us and how important it is to minimize stress with regular exercise, nutritious food, and a good support system. Your genes may make you more prone to visible signs of stress, which you don't have much control over. However, you do often have a say in how to deal with the stress. The examples we discussed in chapter 3 are a great place to start.

- What and how you eat. As you learned in chapter 2, a diet full of fresh and potent nutrients will keep you looking vibrant when a diet of junk food will not. Even yo-yo dieting, which stretches skin, can damage your skin's elasticity, making it droopy. (See this as yet another good reason not to go on a diet, but to eat like the French!)

SMOKING, *MON DIEU!*

When my Parisian friends are stressed, they have a plan. They go to a day spa and have a long, soothing, and skin-firming facial or scrub. Then they'll go out to dinner with their girlfriends and commiserate over a bottle or two of their favorite Bordeaux with their steak and salad. Sounds wonderfully healthy, right?

Add in the pack of cigarettes she'll smoke that day, however, and all her healthy intentions go—literally—up in smoke.

Frenchwomen still smoke way too much. They don't deny it, and they're constantly trying to quit. Sometimes they succeed, but as soon as they gain a pound or two—a common side effect of quitting smoking—back to the lighting up and coughing they go.

I have to say this with a rueful smile because I used to be just like my friends. I started smoking one cigarette a day with my first boyfriend when we were seventeen, and I stopped only when I arrived in New York and the copious restrictions made it nearly impossible (thank goodness!) to smoke anywhere. I'd see other smokers huddled outside their office buildings, in summer's heat or winter's cold or when it was pouring rain. Frenchwomen may smoke a lot, but they are never that desperate for a cigarette that they'd puff away in these conditions.

Plus, of course, I knew how bad even this one-cigarette habit was for my health. I was setting a terrible example for my children, and I don't miss it a bit.

Smokers who try to quit and don't succeed usually know that nicotine is more addictive than heroin, cocaine, and alcohol. They know that if you want to die young and look old, smoking will help you do that. What they often don't know (or want to know) are the terrible particulars.

Smoking reduces 30 percent of your oxygen intake and releases hundreds of toxins into your system, including poisonous gases like carbon monoxide, formaldehyde, hydrogen cyanide, and nitric oxide, as well as toxic substances such as acetone, ammonia, arsenic, benzene, lead, mercury, and tar. Every time you inhale, you're producing carcinogens and free radicals, leading to a cascade of damage, particularly reduced blood flow and oxygen to your cells. Nicotine also blocks estradiol, a form of estrogen in the skin, leaving it drier and thinner. It degrades collagen while causing its production to drop and makes you even more susceptible to sun damage. And as smoking inhibits healing and causes bleeding during surgery, smokers are at greater risk for postsurgical complications.

This explains why smokers often develop deep wrinkles, leathery skin, and a grayish tinge to their skin long before nonsmokers of the same age. In addition, long-term smokers are up to four times more likely to turn prematurely gray, and they're more than twice as likely to lose their hair than nonsmokers.

They are also at a higher risk for skin cancer, particularly squamous cell cancer, in addition to lung, throat, and mouth cancers. Melanoma, the most lethal form of skin cancer, also tends to kill smokers more quickly than nonsmokers, due to their compromised immune systems.

Still want to light up?

WHY DOES SKIN AGE?

If we knew what turns on the aging process, we'd know how to turn it off!

Every day, your skin is assaulted on the outside from the elements and from the inside by its own energy production process. Your skin and body age not just from the stresses of life in the twenty-first century but also because, every second of our turbocharged day, tiny invisible aggressors called free radicals are on the attack.

FREE RADICALS AND OXIDATION
Aging Inside Our Bodies

As our cells age, they don't replicate as effectively as they once did; furthermore, they can replicate only fifty times before they cease to function. This predetermined expiration date is called cellular senescence. When your collagen and elastin cells approach their senescence, you'll suffer a loss of firmness, resilience, and vibrancy. Stress or shock can hasten cellular senescence, which explains why suffering from a tragedy or even a very bad sunburn can make you look older seemingly overnight.

Free radicals are inescapable, as they're the by-products of your body's energy production process. A free radical is defined as a molecule with an unpaired electron; since it's missing its pair, it becomes wildly unstable, desperately seeking out its other half. It finds one by attacking other molecules in an effort to snitch one of their electrons in an endless cycle. The result is cell damage and ultimate breakdown, leading to aging.

Free radicals are also responsible for oxidizing your skin.

Oxidation is a simple and unavoidable natural process. It causes apples to turn brown, cars to rust, butter to go rancid, and your skin to age prematurely. In fact, oxidation is responsible for dull, blah skin as well as an astonishing four out of five wrinkles—because it affects the skin's levels of collagen and elastin that keep it looking plump and youthful.

Luckily, recent research has uncovered ways to slow down oxidation naturally. In fact, this is the same research I mentioned in the introduction to this book—the studies that have demonstrated the role of polyphenols, the anti-aging compounds found in certain foods, especially grapes and other foods that are red, purple, and blue (like plums and blueberries), and inspired Bertrand and me to launch Caudalie. Chapter 5 shows how this groundbreaking research can help you turn back the hands of time.

Aging Outside Our Bodies

Free radicals are generated by anything toxic that you inhale or ingest, such as pollution and cigarette smoke; fried, barbecued, processed, and junk food; furniture polish and paint; or petroleum-based products.

Fortunately, you can fight these environmental assaults by following the suggestions in this book. You can easily do this with daily, comprehensive sun protection; by not smoking or drinking too much; and by eating nutritious, fresh food loaded with nutrients.

And by using antioxidants. Antioxidants—hence their name—fight oxidation. They're molecules, both natural and manmade, that can prevent or slow down the cellular damage caused by free radicals. The goal of antioxidants is to block the production of free radicals and facilitate your cells' natural defense process.

The sooner you start tackling free radicals—preferably before you're thirty, when the effects really start to show—the sooner you'll see results and the less you'll age as time goes on. (One caveat: Smokers need medical advice from their physician about how to use antioxidant supplements, as excessive doses may lead to the opposite results, especially for heavy smokers.)

HORMONES AND SKIN AGING

As women age, their hormone levels naturally begin to decline. Perimenopause is the stage, usually taking place over several years in our late forties to early fifties, where these hormonal fluctuations often have noticeable symptoms. Eventually, when the female hormones have declined to a point where a woman hasn't menstruated for a year, she's considered to be menopausal.

Some women breeze through perimenopause, while others struggle with hot flashes, night sweats, depression, mental fog, concentration lapses, mood swings, weight gain, anxiety, and insomnia. Skin can be noticeably affected, too, as it becomes thinner and drier. Because the feminizing hormones are in decline, the masculinizing hormones can become dominant. Hair often thins where you already have it and can sprout where it's least wanted, usually on or under your chin or around the lips.

Women with symptoms that affect their quality of life and health need to consult their gynecologists for options. Hormone replacement therapy (HRT), usually a combination of estrogen and progesterone, used to be readily prescribed but is controversial due to a long-term study showing that there may be an elevated risk of heart attacks, strokes, blood clots, and breast cancer for women who took HRT for a number of years. These risks are small, but you need to make an informed choice. Supplemental estrogen definitely improves your skin's moisture content and vibrancy, and it has other health benefits as well.

THE NUMBER ONE SECRET TO PREVENT AGING

It's called sun damage.

Like many beauty trends of the past century, we have Coco Chanel to thank (or blame) for our love of the sun. She threw away the parasols and gloves and hats that women had used for centuries to protect their skin and basked in the hot sunshine of Provence.

Because of Chanel, not to mention the Hollywood stars who constantly glowed from the California sunshine, suddenly, tanning became *de rigueur.* No longer was tanned skin a sign that a woman had been outside working in the fields all day. It was "healthy." It was modern. It was attractive.

My mother's generation was so obsessed with tanning that, before tanning oil was available, they resorted to their own means. My mother and her friends would go begging to the farms up in the mountains and ask for some of the grease the farmers used on their cows' udders to aid in the milking process. That was a primitive precursor to tanning oil, and it didn't smell anywhere as delicious as Bain de Soleil.

Like Chanel, I love basking in the warm Provençal sun. But I also know it wreaks havoc on my skin.

There really is no such thing as a "healthy" tan. Any changes to your skin tone due to UV radiation means you have taken a solar sledgehammer to your collagen and elastin as well as damaged your cellular DNA. If you've gotten a burn, you can see the damage. If you haven't, the damage is invisible—but it can last forever.

Worse, it can kill you, which is why the US Department of Health and Human Services includes UV radiation on its list of known carcinogens.

When you got a tan when you were a child or young adult, your tan lines eventually disappeared, didn't they? Same thing with that adorable smattering of freckles on your nose you got when you went to summer camp. They faded as soon as the leaves started to fall. But when you reach a certain age, the tan lines won't go away and the freckles won't fade. You might even notice reverse freckles, which are white spots, or other discolorations causally known as age spots. Or you might notice other dark spots, dryness, roughness, precancerous lesions, wrinkles, fine lines, deep furrows, visible blood vessels, growths, skin cancer—it's all sun damage, properly called photoaging.

The damage caused by sun exposure accumulates over time. Even if you can't see the damage yet or even if you don't slather yourself in oil and spend hours tanning on a hot day, no one is immune to UV radiation and its devastating effects.

Down in the dermis, this is what you can't see:

- Sun damages melanocytes, the cells that produce pigment, which is why you see the hyperpigmentation spots on your skin.

- Blood vessels become thinner, so you're more likely to bruise easily.

- Free radicals develop, which damage your skin's collagen and elastin framework, leaving your skin less resilient.

- Sun exposure can also alter the function of the Langerhans cells that help maintain your body's immunity to infections. Overexposure to UV radiation may suppress proper functioning of your immune system and your skin's natural defenses. This may explain why you got a cold (or a cold sore) when you were baking on a Hawaiian beach during your long-awaited vacation.

UV RADIATION

Sun exposure is so damaging because of ultraviolet radiation, or UV.

Ultraviolet light is classified by wavelengths (nanometers, or nm) into three types: UVA (400–320 nm), UVB (320–290 nm), and UVC (290–200 nm). The shorter the wavelength and the lower the number, the greater the energy level of the light. UVC radiation could kill us, but fortunately it's absorbed in the atmosphere and never reaches the ground.

I wish I could say the same about UVB and UVA rays. They're ever present, which is why you can get a horrific sunburn on a gloomy, cloudy day.

UVA—*A* Is for the Aging Ray

UVA rays penetrate with a terrible efficiency down into the deepest layers of your skin, where it damages your DNA, collagen, and elastin and stimulates production of the pigment-producing melanocytes responsible for hyperpigmentation and uneven skin tone. It causes cancer, particularly melanoma.

The big problem with UVA is that it's always out there, in much higher amounts than UVB. Not even glass windows can prevent you from exposure. If your sunscreen isn't broad-spectrum, you won't have any protection against it, either.

UVB—*B* Is for the Burning Ray

UVB rays literally "cook" the surface of the skin, destroying cellular DNA and releasing free radicals. Excessive exposure can create abnormal skin cells, which can lead to precancerous lesions and skin cancers. As you likely know, UVB rays are strongest between 10:00 A.M. to 4:00 P.M., especially in summer months and in areas closer to the equator. At least UVB doesn't penetrate glass.

Note: Whenever you get a prescription, ask your doctor if it causes sensitivity to UV exposure. If so, you can get rashes, irritation, and increase your risk of a bad sunburn. Antifungals, antihistamines, antimicrobials, antiseptics, coal tar, contraceptives, dyes, nonsteroidal anti-inflammatory drugs (NSAID), perfumes and essential oils, sulfa drugs, tetracycline, and tricyclic antidepressants put you most at risk.

Protect yourself at all times from the sun—not just when you're going to the beach or lying out in the backyard for a little bit of a tan. Even if you're outdoors only to walk to your car and then to your office, you still need to protect yourself. Get into the daily habit of putting your sunscreen or protective clothing on in the morning, before you leave the house. And don't forget your neck, hands, legs, or any other exposed part of your body. You won't see any visible difference tomorrow, but you certainly will a few years from now. Don't let these invisible changes happen when they're so easily prevented!

Skin Cancer Can Kill You

According to the Centers for Disease Control and Prevention (CDC), the death rate from melanoma in the United States has been going up about 4 percent a year since 1973—and these rates are increasing more rapidly than for any other cancer. Even more worrisome, skin cancer is the most common type of cancer in America—one in five Americans will develop skin cancer in their lifetime, with about 65 percent of melanomas and 90 percent of basal and squamous cell skin cancers attributed to UV exposure. The good news is that it's the easiest to prevent.

There are three types of skin cancers:

- Basal cell cancers are the most common, appearing as small, fleshy bumps or nodules, often on the head and neck. They grow slowly and rarely spread, but if untreated can penetrate into bones.

- Squamous cell cancers appear as nodules or as red, scaly patches. The tumors can grow very large and spread into different parts of the body.

- Melanoma is the deadliest skin cancer because it easily metastasizes, spreading all over your body. It can appear anywhere, even on areas that don't get regular sun exposure. Some people will develop it even if they've had minimal sun exposure over the years, the same way that nonsmokers can develop lung cancer.

Tanning booths are especially risky, as the sunlamps are pure UVA. Worse, sometimes they aren't well adjusted, which contributes to an even higher high dose of UVA exposure. They won't burn you, of course (only UVB can do that), but their intensity will definitely damage your cells deep in the dermis and below.

DR. WALDORF'S BEAUTY SECRET FOR AGING WELL

I asked my friend Dr. Heidi Waldorf, a leading New York City dermatologist, for her best anti-aging advice:

"What is the biggest misperception my patients have about skincare? Women often erroneously believe that since there are now so many noninvasive rejuvenation procedures that are a fast, easy, and relatively inexpensive way to erase any skin damage that they don't have to worry about going in the sun or taking proper care of their skin. Yes, lasers, fillers, and peels can do marvels—up to a point. If the damage is deep, surgery might be the only cure. Or—there might be no cure at all.

"Women who do best are those who start a good skincare regimen when they are young, using over-

> the-counter or prescription cosmeceuticals, never failing to use sunscreen, and then gradually progressing on to more intense procedures if and as they need them, rather than waiting for things to fall. That way, with a deft touch, they will look rejuvenated and age-appropriate without needing or wanting more drastic surgical interventions."

ABOUT SUNSCREEN

The French are different from the Americans when it comes to sun worship, as we want to be tan but we don't want to bake in the sun. So we put SPF 50 on our faces, SPF 30 on our bodies, and we can be thoroughly guilty of abusing bronzers as well as self-tanners. (That's why Caudalie created Divine Legs—a gentle bronzer for your legs that doesn't look fake, but smoothes out your color, no matter what your skin tone.) Like many American women, we think that a tan makes you look sexy, healthy, and skinnier. Silly? *Mais, oui!* About to change anytime soon? *Non, non, non!*

We know we're supposed to use sunscreen, so why is skin cancer on the rise? Probably because most people wear sunscreen only when they know they're "going to be in the sun," perhaps during their leisurely Sunday stroll in the park. The problem for your skin is that *every* day is Sunday.

Just as it's hard to educate young women about sun exposure, it is hard to educate them about the proper use of sunscreen. Fortunately, our French pharmacies do a better job than our American counterparts, in part because they change what they carry based on seasonal needs. Pharmacists distribute brochures and handouts to their customers and encourage them to try any new sunscreens. This is not only smart business—it's smart health maintenance.

HOW TO USE SUNSCREEN

Sunscreen was created to keep harmful UVA and UVB rays from penetrating into your skin. When a sunscreen is labeled as broad spectrum, its active ingredients absorb most UVB and UVA and prevent them from reaching the skin, in the same way that the molecules of the atmosphere absorb UVC and prevent it from reaching the ground.

There are two types of sunscreen agents: chemical blockers that absorb ultraviolet light, and physical blockers that reflect ultraviolet light back into the environment.

The most common UVA chemical blockers are meradimate, avobenzone (Parsol 1789), and Mexoryl. The most common UVA physical blocker is zinc oxide.

The most common UVB and UVA chemical blockers are ensulizole, octinoxate, homosalate, octisalate, octocrylene, oxybenzone, Padimate O, titanium dioxide, and Tinosorb (which is not FDA-approved but is available in Europe).

An SPF can refer only to UVB ray blocking and is a rough guide for estimating how long you can be out in the sun without getting burned. If you are very fair, for example, and burn in ten minutes on a hot summer's day, SPF 15 will provide fifteen times additional protection. Against this ten minutes of burning, this equals 150 minutes, or two and a half hours. Sunscreen should have a minimum 30+ SPF for sport or outside activities. For daytime wear, most people can use 15 to 30.

Keep in mind, however, that SPF ratings are determined in laboratory conditions, when the correct amount is applied on the testers, and they aren't moving around or sweating or rubbing their faces. This explains why we rarely get the SPF protection we think we're getting—because we don't use enough of it.

For proper protection, you should use a teaspoon of sunscreen *just* for your face. That's a *lot*. If you're planning to be at the beach, apply at least an ounce of sunscreen on the rest of your body, and reapply it every two hours once you get outside. That's a *lot*. If you're just going outside for your regular routine that doesn't involve a lot of sun exposure, you don't need that much, obviously—but if you're swimming or sweating, you do.

Keep this in mind if you like to wear foundation with an SPF. It will actually give you very little protection because you use it sparingly. (Also wearing an SPF 15 foundation with an SPF 15 sunscreen will not give you an SPF 30 sunscreen.) Apply a sunscreen first, let it fully absorb into your skin, and then apply foundation. Any skincare products intended for nighttime use should never include an SPF.

I've found that the best sunscreens have a combination of mineral and chemical blockers. Use an SPF of at least 20. Apply it at least thirty minutes before you leave the house, and reapply it often. Put some on before you leave the office for lunch. If you're swimming or sweating, apply it every hour.

One of the biggest sunscreen mistakes is forgetting to use it not just on your face but all over, especially on your neck and décolleté. In French pharmacies, sunscreen ads and information almost always target all parts of your body. In America, however, products not aimed just at the face don't sell as well, so you don't see them highlighted. You certainly don't want your face to be unlined and young looking while your neck and hands are wrinkled, spotted, and wizened. More important, you don't want to promote a potentially lethal melanoma.

In Europe, where sunscreen regulations are different, any

sunscreen with an SPF, which as you know is only for UVB protection, must contain UVA protection that is at least one-third of the SPF.

If you really don't like sunscreen or don't think you're disciplined enough to apply it as often as needed, be like the French and get yourself a chic, broad-brimmed sun hat. The more *fantastique,* the more you're likely to wear it. Let it become one of your signature looks.

SELF-TANNERS

Self-tanners are great. They contain an FDA-approved color additive, a sugar called dihydroxyacetone (DHA), and it merely tints the dead cells on the surface of your skin, which is why they fade away as these skin cells slough off. Self-tanners usually last from a few days to up to a week.

It's best to do a gentle exfoliation and then moisturize your skin well before applying any DHA-containing product. If your skin is dry or has any unevenly pigmented or rough spots, the color can be blotchy or streaked. As with every skincare product, though, you don't want to overdo it. Start out gently and gradually build up color.

DHA is a safe molecule for external use. Remember, self-tanners have no UV protection if there are no filters in the formula.

DO YOU NEED A DERMATOLOGIST?

The French may not follow the sterling example of Americans who see their dentists twice a year for cleanings and checkups, but this is an essential part of maintaining healthy teeth. But how many of us go to the dermatologist for regular checkups?

Dermatologists are experts at assessing your level of risk, es-

French Beauty Secret

It is very difficult to maintain a milky-white complexion, as it shows every little spot and blotch. What can help is to put a pea-size dab of self-tanner in your daily moisturizer. I often do that when I want a hint of color in my face. You can also include a pea-size dab in your body cream. Experiment with how much you need, as it will depend on how tan you already are and how tanned you want to look. If you are already tan, a bit of self-tanner or a product like Caudalie's Divine Legs will give you a golden hue.

pecially if you have any moles. They'll be able to tell if your skincare regimen is working well and get you on a better one if needed. They can also help you stop yo-yoing between different treatments and products. Instead of needing to see a doctor when your skin is bad, you'll be taught how to cleanse, exfoliate, and hydrate properly so you won't be stripping the necessary oils of your skin, adding years to your appearance.

According to Dr. Waldorf, you should see a dermatologist for any of the following:

- For a baseline, healthy checkup at any age. Your doctor will photograph your entire body and use this in the future for comparison to see if any moles or spots are growing or changing. Given how prevalent skin cancer is, you can't be too safe. Some women go to medi-spas to have moles removed, but this can be risky as the people working there are often not medically trained and can't tell the difference between skin cancer and a benign mole. The same risks go for at-home devices. When it comes to your skin, it's always good to trust a professional.

- If you have any moles, spots, or splotches that don't heal, change shape or color, or appear suddenly and don't go away no matter what you try. A normal pimple doesn't last for months, and scrubbing at it won't make it go away and can make it much worse.

- If you suddenly develop any skin condition such as acne, psoriasis, eczema, painful irritation, or rashes.

- If the texture of your skin changes dramatically. This can be due to fluctuating hormone levels.

- If you start losing a lot of hair on your head or growing it on your face. This, too, might be caused by hormonal changes.

- If you just want advice about more intensive skincare treatments, especially to treat sun damage.

SUN EXPOSURE AND VITAMIN D

Your body needs vitamin D for the absorption of calcium and for many other crucial functions. Very few foods contain it—except for fatty fish, fish oil, beef liver, cheese, tofu, mushrooms, and eggs (but not in sufficient amounts)—so vitamin D is added to many foods that are part of the typical American diet, like milk and breakfast cereals. In addition, your body can create vitamin D only after sun exposure, which is why it can be difficult to ensure proper levels, especially during winter months and for those who live in northern climates and who rarely spend any time outdoors.

Vitamin D is one of the most necessary of all the vitamins, and many people don't know they're deficient; only a blood test can tell you accurately. You need it to be able to process calcium and keep your bones strong, and low levels can cause immune problems, heart diseases, cognitive impairment, among other issues. Discuss which supplement and levels are best for you with your physician. Look for vitamin D_3 as opposed to D_2, which is better absorbed by your body, and it is more efficient if taken in a supplement with vitamin K.

So don't use the ongoing "debate" about needing adequate vitamin D levels to justify not using sunscreen! It's really not a debate because you always need to protect yourself from harmful UV radiation, and the amount of sun you actually need to create vitamin D is very small.

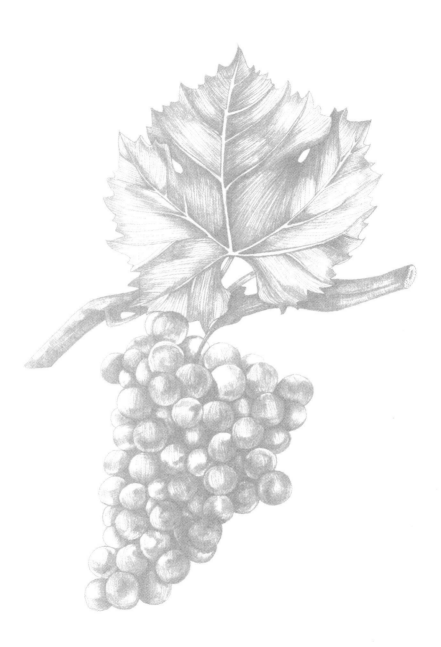

Five

YOUR GUIDE TO SKINCARE INGREDIENTS

Have you ever wondered what those unpronounceable chemicals in your skincare products actually do? Some ingredients might sound complicated or scary when they're nothing more than simple sugar or vitamins. Others, however, can cause irritation, breakouts, and other problems if not adapted to your skin type. For optimal skincare, you need to know what ingredients work best and what to avoid so you can initiate an ingredient detox and start using items that are better for your skin.

Be a smart consumer. You know there's hype in the marketing and the packaging. If you love a product and you think it works, use it and enjoy it, but it's very easy to educate yourself about ingredients that are truly effective and know that you're getting the best value for your investment.

HOW TO DECODE A LABEL

On the back of the box of your skincare products, there are two kinds of listings: The first is the general ingredients, and they are always listed in descending order of concentration. Often, the first ingredient is aqua or water, or a cetyl alcohol, which is a lubricant and thickening agent. Once you get down to the level of 1 percent, skincare companies can list the ingredients in any order they choose.

The second kind of listing is for active ingredients that are considered drugs by the FDA. These are also listed in the general ingredients list, but the FDA requires companies to list them in a separate Drug Facts box. This box will show the name of the ingredient, its concentration, and its purpose. (For what it's worth, you also see this on the box for medicines.)

Sometimes it's best to have the active ingredients at the top of the general ingredients list, as that means they'll be in the product in higher concentrations. But sometimes you don't need (or want) a lot of a certain ingredient in order for it to be effective. For example, there is an optimum amount of effectiveness for the patented, stabilized resveratrol we use in many Caudalie products. If we added more than this amount, it would not be more effective. This is why it can be difficult to know which products touting their expensive active ingredients are actually worth the cost.

THE WORST INGREDIENTS

Before you read about the best skincare ingredients, this list will help narrow down your choices by indicating which ingredients to avoid. Unfortunately, these are very common because they are inexpensive and get the job done—just not in the best possible way. If you can, check to see if the ingredient is plant derived or synthetic. Skincare companies often choose synthetics, as they are less expensive, but plant-derived products are generally more potent.

ANIMAL INGREDIENTS

You really don't want to put any ingredient sourced from a dead animal on your face or body, do you?

APRICOT PITS

Apricot pits are often found in exfoliants and scrubs, but because they tend to be large and coarse, they can cause chronic irritation and make your skin more sensitive as they strip it of much-needed hydration. This creates a vicious cycle of dryness and breakouts that are then attacked with ever-stronger scrubs to allegedly calm inflamed skin. Even if your skin is very oily, your exfoliant should be as gentle and soft as possible.

BENZOYL PEROXIDE

Available only as a prescription drug in Europe, benzoyl peroxide is extremely irritating, so it's available over the counter only in nail polish. Yet this is one of the most common ingredients in American products that treat acne because it kills the *P. acnes* bacteria and dries out skin. If you find it helps your acne and isn't irritating, use it in concentrations of 2.5 percent or less, but always consult a dermatologist before self-treating. And make sure to massage it into your skin and let it dry completely because it can bleach fabrics.

HYDROQUINONE

This bleaching/lightening agent is commonly used in most American over-the-counter lightening and brightening products, but it's banned in Europe and Asia. Why is it still used here? Because it's extremely effective. However, if you don't use it properly, you can unwittingly overbleach your skin, leaving it mottled and uneven—and the damage is irreparable. Many consumers also think that if a little works, a lot will work even more quickly, and then the damage is done. In addition, large doses of hydroquinone can be carcinogenic. If you do want to use it, do so only under supervision by your dermatologist, and start with the lowest possible concentration.

MINERAL OIL AND PETROLEUM JELLY (VASELINE)

Derived from petrochemicals, mineral oil is found in many skin-care products, usually second on the ingredient list, because it is an extremely inexpensive moisturizer. But any mineral oil product can be comedogenic, meaning that it clogs pores, so there's no reason to use them when so many plant oils are more effective and are far less likely to give you acne.

PHTHALATES

Phthalates are very scary chemical compounds as they can be absorbed by your body, either through your skin or inhalation. Despite the fact that numerous studies have shown them to cause damage to internal organs like your liver, kidneys, lungs, and the female reproductive system, causing sterility, they are still used in cosmetics because they cause "cling," allowing products to last longer when you put them on your skin or hair. This accounts for their use in some nail polishes, hair sprays and gels, deodorants, and perfumes. They can also be found in product packaging to make plastics softer and more pliable.

PRESERVATIVES: FORMALDEHYDE AND PARABENS

Formaldehyde

Formaldehyde is a strong chemical used to build walls and furniture. It's also used in lipstick, deodorant, and nail polish, which is dangerous as it's a known carcinogen and can make you very sick. There is no reason whatsoever for it to be in any skincare product when there are so many other healthy alternatives. Some preservatives (diazolidinyl urea, for example) are also known to release formaldehyde and should be avoided.

Parabens

Parabens have been used for decades as preservatives in a wide range of products. They're popular because they are effective, cheap, and easy to use. And they kill possible contaminates, meaning they can assure a long shelf life.

But some parabens disrupt your endocrine system and thereby affect hormone function. They have literally been found in breast tumors. Because of this, I do not use any parabens.

Five parabens have been banned in Europe: isopropyl, isobutyl, phenyl, benzyl, and pentyl paraben. It isn't easy to replace them with food-grade preservatives (which is what Caudalie and many other cosmetics companies do), but it's an effective alternative. In addition, the best way to preserve cosmetics and keep them free from contamination is to put them in a tube instead of a jar.

SODIUM LAURETH SULFATE

Want to wash the grime-encrusted wheels of your car? Choose a detergent that's chock-full of sulfates, because they make lots of foam and suds and get the job done quickly. But you certainly don't want to put such harsh cleansers on your hair or skin. You don't need foaming bubbles for clean hair, so avoid any product with sodium laureth sulfate or sodium lauryl sulfates.

THE VERY BEST SKINCARE INGREDIENTS

Now that you know what to avoid, here's what works best. There are three categories: natural and essential oils; natural (plant-derived) and synthetic (biotech-created) ingredients; and my favorite category, polyphenols.

NATURAL OILS ARE GREAT FOR YOUR SKIN

One of the great fallacies of skincare is that oily skin or skin prone to breakouts should never be touched with oil. *Au contraire*—when you use the right kind of oil on your skin and keep it properly hydrated, oil production in your sebaceous glands actually *decreases*. That's why Frenchwomen love to use oils to cleanse, moisturize, and treat their skin whenever possible, and you can easily do the same.

Oils are a fantastic addition to your skincare arsenal. Not only are they easy to find and highly effective, but they're also inexpensive and safe.

When you are choosing an effective oil-based cleanser, moisturizer, or serum, realize that there are two kinds of oils to use: plant-based oils that are therapeutic and the base for your products; and essential oils, which are distilled essences of plants (herbs, flowers, trees, roots, etc.) that are also therapeutic as well as highly concentrated and so should be used sparingly. Oils are found in over-the-counter products, or in homemade products that contain, for example, grape-seed, avocado, apricot, borage, evening primrose, sweet almond, or jojoba oil. (You'll see examples in the recipes in chapter 8.)

1. PLANT OILS

Plant oils are extracted from plants either by pressing the seeds or by macerating the seeds and roots. Different plant oils all have different properties, and the best are non-comedogenic, easily absorbed by your skin, and laden with essential fatty acids that are extremely nourishing. Most of these oils have no scent.

Apricot Oil

Apricot oil is extracted from the apricot kernel and rarely feels greasy on your skin. It's especially soothing for dry skin.

Used in: Body creams, moisturizers.

Argan Oil, Extra-virgin and Organic

You probably know that argan oil is great for your hair, but it's also wonderful on skin. Argan trees grow in the south of Morocco, and their hard-hulled fruits contain kernels that are cold-pressed to extract the oil. Argan oil has an exceptionally high content of unsaturated fatty acids and linoleic acid to keep skin hydrated.

Used in: Body oils, hair oils, face oils, body scrubs.

Avocado Oil

As with all vegetable oils, avocado oil is rich in unsaturated fatty acids, especially in oleic acid, which explains why it penetrates so easily and effectively into your skin.

Used in: Body creams, hand creams, hair oils, masks, moisturizers, eye creams.

Borage Oil

This oil is rich in gamma linoleic acid (omega-6), giving it soothing and smoothing properties ideal for those with sensitive skin.

Used in: Body creams, moisturizers.

Coriander Oil

Coriander is native to southern Europe. Its oil is extracted and refined from selected seeds. Its exceptional petroselenic acid (omega-12) content makes it an ideal moisturizer for dry and damaged skin. It also carries active ingredients into the heart of skin cells.

Used in: Anti-aging products, face oils.

Grape-seed Oil

My favorite oil, this priceless treasure from the vine is extracted from grape seeds and refined. At Caudalie, it takes 110 pounds of grape seeds to produce only one liter of oil. That's a lot of grapes!

Grape-seed oil is nongreasy, so its dry finish makes it ideal for all skin types, and it contains high levels of linoleic acid (omega-6, an essential fatty acid, as you learned in chapter 2) and vitamin E. As a result, it's an excellent antioxidant that regenerates, nourishes, and restructures even the driest skin.

Used in: Body creams, cleansers, hair oils, body oils, face oils, scrubs, masks, moisturizers.

Hibiscus Oil

Hibiscus is also known as the "flower of eternity." Its oil is extracted by cold-pressing the seeds, which contain large amounts of unsaturated fatty acids that are protective and hydrating like those of argan oil.

Used in: Body oils, hair oils, face oils, body scrubs, eye creams.

Jojoba Oil

Nicknamed "desert gold," jojoba is a shrub from the desert regions of Arizona and Mexico. Jojoba oil has been used for skincare for more than a hundred years, due to its biocompatibility with skin.

It's also soothing, softening, and regenerating and prevents dehydration without leaving any oily residue, making it ideal for those with acne-prone skin.

Used in: Balancing and moisturizing products, face oils.

Musk Rose

Musk rose contains enough fatty acids (omega-3 and -6) and vitamin A to regenerate new cells while revitalizing young cells. It's also good for wrinkle prevention.

Used in: Moisturizers, face oils.

Prickly Pear Oil

The prickly pear is a thorny plant native to Mexico. Its oil, obtained by cold-pressing the seeds, is rich in linoleic acid and also known for its brightening properties and ability to protect your skin from UVA rays.

Used in: Anti-aging, antioxidant, and whitening face oils.

Sandalwood Kernel Oil

Sandalwood oil is extracted from the nut of the plant that grows in India, Nepal, Australia, and Hawaii. It's rich in oleic acid (omega-9 fatty acid), which gives an instant wrinkle-smoothing effect, and ximenynic acid (omega-7 fatty acid), used to treat eczema.

Used in: Anti-aging products, face oils.

Sesame Oil

Produced from sesame seeds, sesame oil is rich in monounsaturated and polyunsaturated fatty acids. This nourishing oil is nongreasy and particularly suitable for dry skin, acts effectively against flakiness, and protects the skin from external aggressions.

Used in: Body oils, hair oils, face oils, body scrubs.

Sweet Almond

This oil is famed for penetrating deep into your cells, where it gives radiance to dull, tired, or stressed-out skin.

Used in: Moisturizers, face oils.

ARE OIL-FREE PRODUCTS GOOD TO USE, ESPECIALLY FOR ACNE?

Now that you know that oils are good for your skin, even if you tend to be oily and/or have acne, you don't need to avoid them as you may have done in the past. If you're still worried about oils for whatever reason (maybe you don't like how they feel), however, be warned: The FDA has no specific rules regulating claims that a product is oil-free, so it's hard to know what an oil might be replaced with. A good compromise, especially if you're worried about breakouts, is to try products that contain antibacterial essential oils, especially balm mint, catnip, lavender, lemon, lemongrass, melissa, rosemary, sage, or tea tree, as these oils are highly concentrated and only a very small amount is needed.

---

2. ESSENTIAL OILS

As you learned in chapter 3, essential oils are the distilled essences of different herbs and flowers, containing the volatile aroma compounds of these plants. They are extracted from seeds, bark, stems, roots, leaves, flowers, and/or fruit. They're called "essential" inasmuch as they contain the "essence" of the plant's fragrance and therapeutic components, which become highly concentrated during the distillation process. The composition of any essential oil is very complex; sometimes there are more than one hundred different molecules in it, which is why it smells so wonderful and can have such a powerful effect.

It's also why essential oils should *never* be put directly on your skin or scalp, but mixed in with an unscented plant oil or combination of oils or a cream. (They are not soluble in alcohol or in water.) Make your mixtures, label them, and keep them in dark glass bottles with droppers; you'll need to use only a few drops of the mixture at a time.

You already know how important fragrance has always been to me, and I can indulge my love for it whenever I use an essential oil. Know what to use, and you can instantly create your own wonderful potions as I do. In fact, when my skin is stressed or dry, especially after I've been traveling a lot and the plane air has taken its toll, I'll use one of my oil blends, under my moisturizer before bed and let it work its magic as I sleep. This gives me a super-rich night treatment. Sometimes I'll add twenty drops underneath any treatment mask to intensify its effect. In addition, a few drops of one of my oil blends in a tinted moisturizer or in your foundation will make you look extra-dewy.

These are my favorite essential oils:

Carrot
Carrot oil purifies the skin and removes toxins, organic residues, and pollution. It also helps to renew skin cells.

Used in: Detox and balancing oils.

Lavender
Lavender oil is often used to calm, soothe, and relax. Its properties are anti-inflammatory and healing. I've yet to meet anyone

who doesn't find this scent to be calming and uplifting (and delicious!).

Used in: Detox and balancing oils.

Lemongrass or Lemon Balm

The oils are best for draining, decongesting, and anticellulite.

Used in: Balancing and slimming oils.

Neroli

A common component of many fine perfumes, neroli is distilled from orange blossoms. It has soothing and rebalancing benefits and is helpful for regular, restful sleep, so it's wonderful for your body and your skin when you're exhausted. Even sensitive skin tolerates it well, and it has a skin-cell renewal effect, can help brighten dark spots, and is very soothing.

Used in: Detox oils.

Palmarosa

Palmarosa, grown in India and Vietnam, is also known as the Indian geranium. It belongs to the lemongrass family and is frequently used in traditional Indian medicine. It's wonderful for cell renewal stimulation, moisturization, and healing.

Used in: Moisturizing oils.

Peppermint (*Mentha piperita*)

Peppermint is distinguished from other types of mint by stronger and shorter leaves and a peppery flavor. It's especially refreshing not only to smell but also to tone and wake up your skin.

Used in: Firming oils.

Petitgrain

Petitgrain is extracted from the leaves and twigs of the bitter orange plant. It is a calming and balancing anti-inflammatory that revitalizes your skin. It's especially good for skin that is stressed.

Used in: Detox oils.

Rose

Rose essential oil is extracted from petals by steam distillation. Four *tons* of petals are needed to obtain one kilo (about 2.2 pounds) of essential oil. It is particularly soothing and excellent for treating redness and rosacea, as it's highly tolerated by sensitive and extra-sensitive skin.

Used in: Moisturizing oils.

Rosemary

Rosemary is an aromatic wild shrub that grows in the Mediterranean region. It's rich in volatile oils, flavonoids, and phenolic acids, which are antiseptic, antibacterial, and anti-inflammatory. It is also used for its regenerating and antioxidant properties and as a stabilizer for other ingredients.

Used in: Purifying oils and lotions.

White Sandalwood

This type of sandalwood oil has purifying properties, as it soothes nervous tension and promotes relaxation. It also eliminates dirt, irritation, and inflammation as well as relieves congestion.

Used in: Sensitive skin oils.

3. NATURAL AND SYNTHETIC INGREDIENTS

In addition to the oils listed above, these clinically proven ingredients are top notch as well as the safest I recommend. Some are natural, and others, like ceramides, hyaluronic acid, and peptides (such as Matrixyl), are biotech compounds created in laboratories.

Cassia angustifolia

Cassia is a plant rich in polysaccharides that grows in India and has a strong hygroscopic property, meaning that it absorbs moisture. It has a visible moisturizing effect soon after you put it on, leaving your skin soft and supple.

Used in: Anti-aging products, moisturizers.

Ceramides

Ceramides are moisture-capturing lipids, which means they act as a barrier to keep your skin hydrated.

Used in: Anti-aging products.

Chamomile

Chamomile has been used for centuries in traditional medicines for its soothing, anti-inflammatory properties.

Used in: Sensitive-skin moisturizers.

Fern

Ferns are leafy green plants that contain sugars that form a mesh on the surface of your skin, for an immediate lifting effect.

Used in: Anti-aging, firming products.

Flax

Flax has long been cultivated for its durable yet soft fiber and oil seeds—the ancient Egyptians used flax not only to spin into linen but also in their precious papyrus scrolls. The lignin part of the flax seed is effective at regulating sebum, or oil production. This helps it to reduce oil, refine skin texture, and reduce pore size.

Used in: Moisturizers for oily/acne-prone skin.

Glycolic Acid

One of the family of AHAs, or alpha hydroxy acids, glycolic acid is one of the most common ingredients in skincare products designed to exfoliate. It works by removing the dead skin cells on the top layer of your epidermis, revealing younger and smoother skin underneath.

Used in: Brightening/lightening products, moisturizers for oily/acne-prone skin, pore minimizers.

Hyaluronic Acid

Another very common skincare ingredient, hyaluronic acid is a compound found naturally in your skin. There are two categories of hyaluronic acid: high and low molecular weight (micro). The high molecular weight has an immediate effect of smoothing the skin's surface, while the low weight penetrates for biologically active anti-aging properties. When applied topically, it is a powerful moisturizer that can minimize fine lines and wrinkles.

Used in: Moisturizers (high molecular weight), anti-aging products (low molecular weight).

Imperata cylindrica

This herb can survive in deserts or other arid locations with a high level of salt due to its ability to retain its water content no matter how harsh the outside environment. When used on the skin it is a very powerful and wholly natural moisturizer.

Used in: Moisturizers.

Mango Butter

Mango butter is extracted from the mango kernel and is very similar to shea butter, with emollient and soothing properties.

Used in: Moisturizers.

Olive Squalane

Squalane is an important component of healthy sebum, and it's a great ingredient, as it maintains hydration without being occlusive. It used to be supplied from sharks, but fortunately it is also found in olive oil! It's processed so that it's dry to the touch and nonoily.

Used in: Moisturizers.

Organic Grape Water

Organic grape water is a product unique to Caudalie. This is the vegetable water found in grapes. It is highly mineralized, loaded with vitamins, and has an ideal sugar content to moisturize (+127 percent) the skin and decrease sensitivity (–61 percent).

Used in: Sensitive skin products and moisturizers.

Padinami

An advanced anti-aging extract, it's made from a purified extract of *Padina pavonica* seaweed, a brown algae found in the Mediterranean's temperate waters. When stabilized in jojoba oil, Padinami increases your skin's ability to retain water, making it firmer and improving elasticity.

Used in: Anti-aging, firming products.

Papaya Enzyme (Papain)

Papayas are not only an extremely nutritious fruit, but also wonderfully gentle and natural nonirritating exfoliants. Using them has a near-instantaneous brightening effect, and they also improve your skin's texture.

Used in: Brightening/lightening products, moisturizers for oily/acne-prone skin, pore minimizers.

Peptides and Tetrapeptides

Peptides are lab-created amino acid (the building blocks of protein) molecules with multiple effects. They can stimulate elastin synthesis and improve the structure of elastin fibers, making them a potent fighter against gravity's toll on your skin as well as the loss of elasticity. They can stimulate collagen production and provide hydration, making them wrinkle fighters and moisturizers. And they can have a draining effect that improves your skin's microcirculation, which can help reduce puffiness and dark circles.

There are twenty different amino acids and an infinite variety of peptides, each with different properties. Because they are biotech molecules, they often go by brand names. Caudalie uses the anti-aging, wrinkle-smoothing Dermaxyl CL (palmitoyl oligopeptide and ceramides), the anti-wrinkle Matrixyl 3000 (palmitoyl tetrapetide and tripeptide), and the firming Idealift (acetyl dipeptide cetyl ester), for example, so look at the labels of your skincare products for more details.

Used in: Anti-aging, antisagging, dark circles, eye puffiness, and firming products.

Shea Butter (Fair Trade)

Shea butter is a wonderful emollient and moisturizer with thickening properties, suitable for all skin types, as it is soothing and nonirritating. It is also rich in fatty acids such as linoleic acid and is found in many different skincare products.

Used in: Moisturizers; body, face, and hair oils.

Tannins

Tannins are extracted from the fruit of the Asian tree *Enantia chlorantha*. They have an immediate astringent effect, so they tighten pores and refine skin texture.

Used in: Pore minimizers.

Vinolevure

Vinolevure is a product unique to Caudalie. Extracted from the wine yeast wall, it has a fortifying effect by strengthening your skin's immune function. It also moisturizes deeply.

Used in: Moisturizer and products for sensitive skins.

Vitamin C Ester

When the intrepid explorer Jacques Cartier was snowbound in the Saint Lawrence River in what is now Quebec in 1535, his crew members were dying of scurvy. They knew sailors on long expeditions tended to get this disease, but they had no understanding of its causes or how to cure it. Cartier's crew was saved thanks to a tea the Iroquois tribe native to Quebec made them drink. The tea was made from the bark of a native tree rich in polyphenols and vitamin C.

Vitamin C is necessary not only to prevent scurvy, but also as a potent antioxidant that can boost your skin's radiance and even out your complexion. That's why it's a very common ingredient in many skincare products—but there's a catch. Vitamin C is actually a very fragile molecule, and like resveratrol, if it's not preserved and stabilized properly, it becomes brown and it's basically useless. Make sure you use vitamin C ester, which has been stabilized.

Used in: Anti-aging and antioxidant products.

White Tea

White tea comes from the buds and leaves of the *Camellia sinensis* plant and needs very little processing, so you can utilize all the tea's antioxidant properties.

Used in: Antioxidant moisturizers.

4. POLYPHENOLS

Any time you've bitten into a piece of fruit that you thought was ripe but wasn't, you've come into contact with polyphenols.

Polyphenols are micronutrients, complex molecules that are found in countless plants, primarily fruits and vegetables; legumes, nuts, and seeds; cacao and teas; and, of course, grapes and red wine. Scientists all over the world have extensively studied them for decades, as they have natural antioxidant, antiviral, antibacterial, and antifungal properties and for their many additional health benefits including their skin protectiveness (which I discuss in the section on resveratrol on page 135). These benefits include anti-aging and cancer-fighting properties, improving cardiovascular health (especially blood flow through your arteries) and regulating cholesterol levels, blood sugar regulation (to counter the effects of diabetes), and to normalize blood pressure. They may help lower the risk of neurological conditions such as dementia, Alzheimer's disease, and stroke and diseases like multiple sclerosis. They also boost sirtuins, a class of proteins that enhance the life span of your cells—making them ideal for skincare and protection. I discuss sirtuins more on page 136.

The best fruit sources of polyphenols are apples, apricots, berries (all types), cherries, cranberries, dates, kiwi, lemons, limes, mangoes, nectarines, oranges, peaches, pears, plums and prunes, pomegranates, raisins, grapes, and tangerines.

The best vegetable sources are artichokes, broccoli, celery, cherry tomatoes, corn, eggplant, fennel, leafy greens (all types), onions (all types), parsnips, red cabbage, sweet potatoes, and watercress.

The best legume, nut, and seed sources are dried beans (all types), chickpeas, fava beans, lentils, and peas; ground and tree nuts (all types), especially red-skinned peanuts; and flax, pumpkin, and sunflower seeds.

The best cacao sources are dark chocolate made from at least 60 to 70 percent cacao and raw cacao nibs. The best tea sources are green and black teas.

The best wine source of polyphenols is red wine. The younger the wine, the more polyphenols it contains. Most of a grape's polyphenols are concentrated in the solid parts—the seeds, stems, and skins. They comprise a large family: Resveratrol, Viniferine, and procyanidolic oligomers (PCO) are all polyphenols. The chemical structure of polyphenols is what gives them their antioxidant proprieties.

When wine is being made, the alcohol created by the fermentation process helps extract polyphenols during its contact with the grape seeds and skin. Since this process takes time—approximately eight weeks at Château Smith Haut Lafitte while the wine is in a large vat—a *lot* of polyphenols are extracted. White wine and Champagne contain fewer polyphenols than red wine because the grapes do not macerate during fermentation, so there isn't enough time for the polyphenols to be extracted. Unfortunately, sweet grape juice has few polyphenols because it doesn't undergo a long fermentation process, either.

It's important to know that the potency of food polyphenols depends on their bioavailability, or how well your body can utilize them. Polyphenols can quickly degrade and be rendered basically useless due to oxidation. Food that has been oxidized (such as when an apple slice turns brown when left out) loses valuable micronutrients. Heating or processing food (during canning, for example, or when cooked) also affects polyphenol levels. Eating a handful of grapes or bright purple plums will give you lots of polyphenols; eating a pastry with grape or plum filling will not.

That's why drinking a small glass of red wine each day is an excellent way to add bioavailable polyphenols into your diet; the wine-making process removes polyphenols' natural astringency without affecting their potency. In fact, the power of polyphenols is the primary reason for red wine's much-touted and researched benefits, especially for cardiovascular health. In the well-known Copenhagen City Heart Study, which tracked more than 13,285 men and women over twelve years, those who drank red wine reduced their chances of getting heart disease or a stroke by half compared to those who never drank any wine. Scientists believe that the specific polyphenol found in red wine is one of the primary reasons for these results. That polyphenol is called resveratrol.

RESVERATROL

Resveratrol is a natural substance produced by grapevines to protect them from daily micro-traumas. Scientists have also found that resveratrol is concentrated in grape skins and stalks as a first defense against any fungus that might attack them. (It takes more than one thousand pounds of grape stalks to make only one pound of pure resveratrol!) More than eight hundred scientific articles on resveratrol have been published only in 2014. According to a recent study by the Scripps Research Institute that was reported in *Nature,* one of the most prestigious science journals in the world, this naturally occurring protective factor in grapes is the same kind of factor that allows resveratrol to bind to certain enzymes in your body, enter your cells, and activate your longevity genes as well as cancer-fighting genes.

In other words, the resveratrol in red grapes has been proven to improve the health and life span of your cells. Let's take a look at this remarkable feat in detail:

Anti-aging

When used in skincare products, resveratrol is particularly good at targeting the fibroblasts responsible for the renewal of the collagen and elastin that support your skin's structure. If you'll recall from the last chapter, collagen and elastin naturally degrade as we get older, so keeping your fibroblasts young and healthy helps you maintain youthful and firm skin.

Activates Sirtuins for Anti-aging

Sirtuin is short for silent information regulator two genes, which are found in fetal and adult tissues. They aid in the repair of your DNA and reduce inflammation. Most important, they also appear to hold the keys to human health and longevity—and may, some-day soon, unlock the secrets to slowing down the actual aging process, not just for skin but for your entire body.

Some of the most fascinating research we've been working on has been with Dr. David Sinclair, a professor at Harvard Medical School in the Department of Genetics and codirector of the Paul F. Glenn Laboratories for the Biological Mechanisms of Aging. He is also co–chief editor of the academic journal *Aging* and one of *Time*'s 100 Most Influential People of 2014. He is one of the world's leading experts on sirtuins and is referred to in nearly every study published by his peers in medical literature. I first read about him when an article about one of his studies was published in *Nature*. In it, he said that resveratrol was the best molecule to enhance the life span of cells. Then he appeared on the cover of *Fortune* magazine, discussing how if you want live longer, drink wine! (Dr. Sinclair is originally from Australia, but I think he is secretly French.) We met in September 2013 in Paris when I invited him to the scientific conference on resveratrol that we organized at Caudalie headquarters, and he told me he'd studied hundreds of anti-aging molecules, and resveratrol was by far the most interesting. It was an instant validation of everything Caudalie had been striving to do, and we have since teamed up with him to create skincare products based on his newest research. (We are planning to launch these new products soon.)

Dr. Sinclair's laboratory was the first to show that sirtuins can be activated by small molecules like resveratrol, and that resveratrol has also been shown to activate the genes that fight aging. Such stimulation makes your cells live longer. Here's what's so exciting about the sirtuin/resveratrol connection: The longer your cells live, the less you age. In other words, sirtuins can make you live longer while feeling younger. *Incroyable!*

Antioxidant

You already learned how important it is to use antioxidants to combat the free radicals that cause oxidation. Resveratrol is a natural antioxidant that targets inflammation. Its activities last throughout the average twenty-one-day life span of a skin cell, so during that time it can protect these cells from damage from the sun's UVA radiation. Not only that, but resveratrol also protects cells from UV-induced damage such as collagen degradation.

Antiglycation

Glycation is a reaction between proteins and sugars. This is called the Maillard reaction, and you can see it in your skillet anytime you accidentally overcook your food and it turns brown or burned. Glycation is not a good thing for your skin. Technically speaking, glycation takes place when sugar molecules attach themselves to proteins, leading to irreversible bonds that can make your skin stiff and fragile. This also reduces your skin's ability to regenerate collagen, which provides the underlying support to prevent wrinkles and looseness. Fortunately, resveratrol has the ability to avert glycation-induced damage to your skin's structure by neutralizing the glycation process—this is what prevents the formation of deep wrinkles.

How to Best Use Resveratrol

As you just read, there are two important reasons to use resveratrol. You want to eat polyphenol/resveratrol-rich foods and drink polyphenol/resveratrol-rich tea and red wine for good health and for sirtuin activation from the inside out; and you want to use resveratrol-rich skincare products for good skin from the outside in.

In recent years, resveratrol has started to be sold as a supplement, and this can be beneficial if you're not a red wine drinker. The brand I recommend is Caudalie's Vinexpert grape dietary supplement with grape extract, evening primrose oil, and borage oil.

Resveratrol can be used in much higher concentrations when applied directly to skin than when taken as a supplement, but it's important to know that not all topical products with resveratrol are effective. Resveratrol is an amazingly powerful polyphenol, but it is highly unstable when exposed to air and sunlight, just as vitamin C is. You may have, at some point, bought a skincare product that had vitamin C in it, and after using it for a short time began to notice that the product was turning color. It hadn't spoiled—it had oxidized. Once that happens, the active ingredients have degraded and they are no longer active. This makes the product basically worthless.

When we first met Professor Vercauteren, he had just gotten a patent for polyphenols and was working hard on another one by investigating how to stabilize resveratrol to inhibit the oxidation process. Until he did, no one could claim the resveratrol in any topical product would actually be able to work. Once resveratrol has been stabilized, however, it will not degrade or oxidize, so you can be sure the product will deliver what it promises—a powerful boosting of your collagen and elastin fibers that will refirm your skin and keep it looking youthful.

It took Professor Vercauteren many years to finally figure out how to do this, and once he did, he was able to obtain the patent on it. We realized its value, and its potency is what allowed us to grow our company and be certain that all our resveratrol-containing products would work effectively. Caudalie is the only skincare company that contains stabilized vine resveratrol, as well as the only one that titrates the resveratrol content so we can guarantee a minimum amount of this ingredient in each product (when you see resveratrol 1000 ppm, it means the product contains one thousand parts per million pure resveratrol in a jar of the product). Our resveratrol has been stabilized with a fatty acid so it actually works.

VINIFERINE

It was an ancient tradition in the vineyards of France for the women who worked there during the harvests to rub the sap from the grapevines on their skin. They knew it was a highly effective skin brightener and got rid of any brown spots or freckles. That's what inspired us to study vine sap. Not surprisingly, we found it contains polyphenol molecules that are natural melanin regulators. We were then able to patent Viniferine, based on this sap, a few years later, and it's now the star ingredient in many of our products.

Thanks to its anti-inflammatory properties, Viniferine is sixty-two times more effective than vitamin C to brighten, gently lighten dark spots, and even out skin tone. Even those with the most sensitive skin can use it. Our Vinoperfect Radiance Serum, in which Viniferine is an active ingredient, is our internationally bestselling product—because it really works. It is the number one anti–dark spot product sold in the French pharmacies since 2008.

FRAGRANCE, IRRITATION, AND YOUR PRODUCTS

You may have read in beauty magazines and websites or been told at the cosmetics counters that fragrance, an ingredient found in countless products, is an irritant and potential allergen. But there is a difference between irritation and a true allergy. According to Dr. Waldorf, true allergies aren't very common, and they are more often to chemicals than to fragrance, which is rare. An irritant can cause a negative reaction in *anyone* if they use too much. An allergen, such as to a specific plant oil or chemical, affects only certain people.

Over the years, women have told me that they're becoming more and more reactive to skincare ingredients. Many skincare products have anywhere from ten to twenty different ingredients. Layer a lot of different products on, or use too much of them, and your skin can rebel. If so, it can be hard to figure out what precisely has triggered a reaction. Sometimes, you can be unaware that your favorite products have a new formulation, which might be more irritating; or your skin might also be stressed due to climate or other issues, and it will be more hypersensitive than usual, too.

But, according to Dr. Waldorf, many of her patients who tell her they have sensitive skin don't really have it—they're just using products that are too harsh for them. This can include rough scrubs, some toners with a lot of alcohol, or a strong soap not intended for use on the face. Or, they might not know that they have an underlying skin condition like eczema or rosacea.

Sometimes, reactions might occur because a product has expired. Most products should stay viable for up to three years. Bear in mind that a product in a jar that's applied with your fingers contains more preservatives than products in a tube to prevent degradation from exposure to air. Those with sensitive skin should use products in tubes—and it's also why I try to avoid jars as much as possible. My products are packaged in tubes, pumps, or with droppers except when the viscosity of the formula is too high, making the cream too thick to be placed in a tube.

Still, if any of your skincare products burn, itch, or cause redness, hives, scales, or a rash, you need to see a dermatologist. A patch test can determine whether or not this is an allergy (which can be serious) or simple irritation (which usually goes away with topical treatment). If, for example, you've been using a cream for several months without any problems and then one day it suddenly makes your face extremely red, that is more likely an allergic reaction. Stop using the product and take the container with you to the doctor's office.

There is only a very small amount of fragrance—usually around 0.1 percent of the formula in a serum, because a tiny amount goes a very long way—in our products, and they are hypoallergenic.

Many companies advertise the fact that they're fragrance-free as a selling point, but bear in mind that this drastically limits their choice of effective ingredients.

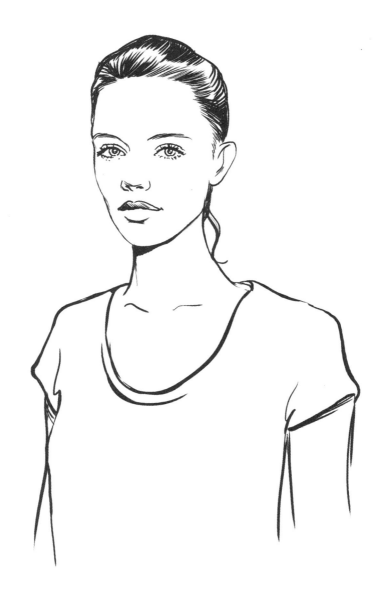

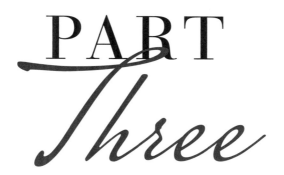

PART
Three

The Essentials of Beautiful,
Healthy Skin

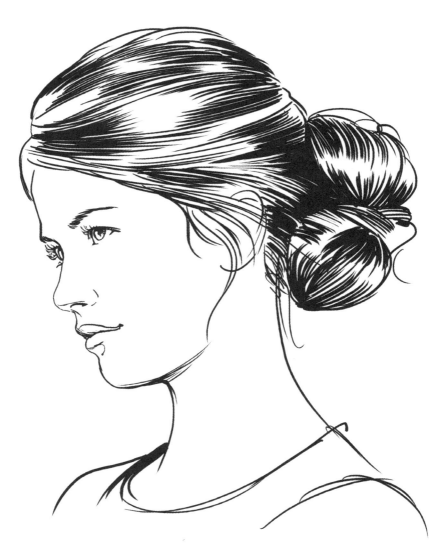

Six

TAKING CARE OF YOUR FACE AND NECK

The first step to having beautiful, healthy skin is to recognize your skin type. Your skin *type* (or what your skin inherently is: normal, dry, oily, sensitive) is different from your skin *condition* (or how your skin feels and looks). This explains why you can have, for example, oily skin with occasional dry patches, or normal skin that is dehydrated because you go swimming in a chlorinated pool several times a week. Once you know your skin type, you can choose the appropriate treatments and products. Bear in mind, of course, that skin types can change over time. Teenage skin tends to be oilier than skin of older women, for example.

HOW TO RECOGNIZE YOUR SKIN TYPE
YOU HAVE DRY OR DEHYDRATED SKIN . . .

If your skin is thin, easily reddened, fragile, and often feels tight and uncomfortable. You also tend to have the following:

- Dry patches

- Dullness

- Fine wrinkles

- Lack of radiance

YOU HAVE NORMAL SKIN . . .

If your skin feels comfortable. It's neither too oily nor too dry, although environmental factors can make it dry or dehydrated. This type is usually found on young women, and you may tend to have the following:

- Occasional breakouts

- Occasional dryness

YOU HAVE OILY OR COMBINATION NORMAL/OILY SKIN . . .

If your skin produces too much sebum. How much sebum, or oil, is produced is largely genetic, although extrinsic factors like the wrong kind of oil-stripping cleanser or heat and humidity can add to the problem. Combination skin refers to the type where the T-zone of your forehead and nose area tends to be oilier than the rest of your face. You tend to have the following:

- Enlarged pores

- Oily or shiny patches, especially in your T-zone

- Pimples and/or blackheads or other skin imperfections

- Shiny skin

- Cheeks that can become dehydrated, even if the rest of your face is oily

ABOUT ACNE

Acne is not caused by eating chocolate or French fries. That's a relief. But for women who suddenly develop acne as adults, it can be devastating to have such visible skin problems. Acne is an inflammatory disease that is caused by genetics, your fluctuating hormone levels, and the *P. acnes* bacteria. These hormonal changes affect how often your skin cells turn over; if they don't turn over as they should—becoming stickier and oilier instead—pores get clogged and pimples and blackheads form.

It's not a good idea to treat acne yourself, especially if it suddenly develops, as this may be an indication of a hormonal imbalance that warrants medical attention from a physician, either your dermatologist or endocrinologist. Over-the-counter acne products are usually targeted to teens that tend to have oilier and less fragile skin than adults, and they can cause irritation and make your skin look even worse. Your dermatologist can devise the right treatment plan and check your hormone levels, too.

YOU HAVE SENSITIVE SKIN . . .

If your skin is highly reactive, and products often set it off. Sensitive skin is tricky, as you may have been born with a predisposition to it, or you might have unwittingly caused sensitivities over the years due to factors such as pollution, extreme climate, smoking, too much sun, your diet, or the kind of skincare products you have used. You also tend to have the following:

- Blushing tendency

- Excessive reaction to climate, cosmetics, and/or stress

- Diffuse redness

- Irritation

- Tingling

ABOUT ROSACEA

Rosacea is not acne, although it's often erroneously called "adult acne." It's a common vascular condition that appears as a flush/blush reaction, usually on your cheeks and nose. There are many triggers for it, including alcohol, anxiety, caffeine, cosmetics, embarrassment, fragrance, exercise, foods, heat, prescription drugs, stress, sunlight, and temperature changes, especially extreme heat or cold.

Rosacea is a progressive condition that is incurable, although there are many treatment options. Using acne products can definitely irritate your skin, so seek advice from your dermatologist. You are especially susceptible to UV radiation, which means that daily sunscreen is an absolute must.

TREATMENT REGIMENS FOR YOUR SKIN TYPE

No matter what your skin type, follow these basic steps:

YOUR DAYTIME TREATMENT REGIMEN

1. CLEANSE your face.

Washing your face may seem like a very simple task, but there is actually an art to it.

You should wash your face twice a day, and follow your cleanser with a moisturizing toner and then your treatment serum and moisturizer.

There are different cleansers for different cleansing habits. Pick the cleanser you like:

- A foaming cleanser rinses with water

- A milky cleanser is removed with a toning lotion

- A micellar cleansing water is clear and has the consistency of water. It contains small particles called micelles that work like miniature sponges, mopping up dirt and makeup while dehydrating. Soak a cotton pad with it and apply to your face (it's also a makeup remover). Repeat until the cotton pad remains clean. There is no need to rinse.

2. TONE your skin.

I've found that many American women think toners are astringent in nature and meant only for those with oily skin. But adding a hydrating toner to your routine takes only seconds and will noticeably improve your skin. A good toner will not strip the skin of its natural oils but instead perfect the cleansing step as well as add moisture to your skin and prepare it for your serum or treatment moisturizer. If your skin is dry or sensitive, look for a toner without alcohol. If your skin is oily, look for a toner with antibacterial ingredients and oil or acne-fighting essential oils.

No matter what your skin type, you might want to try Caudalie's Beauty Elixir as it's both a toner and a serum and contains rose, orange blossom, essential oil of mint, essential oil of melissa, and rosemary, myrrh, and benzoin, a very rich antibacterial blend. Using this Elixir is actually my very best beauty secret. Not a day goes by without me spraying it on to refresh my skin and tighten my pores or fix my makeup.

3. Apply SERUM, if needed.

Serums are usually a more potent and concentrated type of skincare product, with more therapeutic and active ingredients than a moisturizer and with an aqueous texture that can penetrate the skin more quickly. They're a must to protect the vulnerable skin of city dwellers dealing with environmental pollution. You need only a few drops.

As with cleansers, you can use different serums or mix up your own; try using a firming serum in the daytime and a super-hydrating one at night. Be sure to always use a moisturizer or sunscreen afterward, as serums are not moisturizers, and you want to make sure your face will be properly hydrated.

4. Apply MOISTURIZER, if needed.

Moisturizers can have a smoothing and hydrating effect that can make fine wrinkles less noticeable. They either add moisture to the stratum corneum or create a barrier so that your natural moisture doesn't evaporate. They're especially needed in colder months, when dry heat can take its toll on your face indoors, while cold and wind strip it dry outside. Drinking water isn't enough to replace this lost moisture—you need a moisturizer to protect your skin. You'll see which type to choose in the section starting on page 156.

After you determine your skin type and according to your skincare needs, select a treatment moisturizer from the list on page 157. If your skin is not very dry, you don't need a very rich cream. Daytime moisturizers are more for protection, while nighttime moisturizers are for treatment and repair and tend to be richer and contain no SPF.

If your skin starts breaking out, you might be overdoing it. Switch to a more lightweight product and use less of it.

5. Apply SUNSCREEN.

As you learned in chapter 4, you should always choose a broad-spectrum sunscreen with a high SPF to protect from UVA (aging) and UVB (burning) radiation.

6. Apply EYE CREAM.

The skin around your eyes is four times thinner than the rest of the skin on your face. And we blink about 1,200 times every hour, which comes to over 28,000 times each and every day! This naturally creates wear and tear on your skin; in addition, your sleep habits and genetic predisposition can leave you with naturally puffy eyes and dark circles. Eye products are designed for this sensitive area, ophthalmologist-tested so they won't affect your eye function, and usually fragrance-free to be less irritating.

Always apply your eye cream in a full circle around your orbital bone—it's not just for eyelids. Look for one that includes hydrating, antiwrinkle, and firming/antipuffing ingredients and lots of antioxidants.

HOW MUCH SHOULD GOOD
SKINCARE COST?

There is such a huge variation on the pricing of skincare products that it's often difficult to know what to buy—and prices change so often that it's impossible to give an accurate range. Is the product really worth a huge price tag or are you paying more for packaging and advertising? Can great products be found in drugstores?

It's hard for me to advise you about what to purchase, as skincare companies are always changing their formulations, and what I say in this book about their products might be outdated by the time you read it. What I can say is that it's most important to purchase a terrific antioxidant moisturizer and serum for your budget, as they provide the most long-lasting benefits for your skin. Read the labels carefully, and look for products that contain the best ingredients I listed in chapter 5, as you can't go wrong with them. Many brands have excellent products, and if you can shop around online, you can often find discounts. You can also save a tremendous amount of money when you buy large bottles of natural oils, which can be found in health-food stores. They're far less expensive than many body lotions because you need to use only a small amount; a large container of organic coconut oil is only about ten dollars and it should last for months. Their only downside is that they can be very greasy on your skin. All the recipes you'll see in chapter 8 are extremely inexpensive.

If, on the other hand, you like what you're using and it makes your skin look good, don't feel that you have to switch. The only time you should make a change is if your favorite product contains ingredients that are on my must-avoid list. You might end up spending more in the long run on undoing any potential damage.

YOUR NIGHTTIME TREATMENT REGIMEN

1. Always REMOVE EYE MAKEUP.

Your eyes are going to be ultra-sensitive no matter what your skin type, so treat them with care when you remove your eye makeup. Avoid any eye makeup remover with any kind of mineral oil, as they are very irritating and pore-clogging for tender skin. I always recommend using a safe and gentle remover that involves minimal use, especially rubbing or a need to use a lot of product—I like to use cleansing oils that are 100 percent natural. They are the most effective makeup removers. No eye makeup remover should ever sting—if it does, find a different one.

2. CLEANSE your face.

Follow the directions for daytime. (If your makeup remover is also a cleanser for your entire face, you can skip this step.)

3. TONE your skin.

Follow the directions for daytime.

4. EXFOLIATE your skin.

Do this at least once a week, and up to twice a week as you get older and skin cell turnover naturally slows down. See the sidebar below for details.

5. Apply SERUM or an OIL, if needed.

Follow the directions for daytime.

6. Apply MOISTURIZER.

Follow the directions for daytime. Do *not* use a moisturizer with an SPF, as it will only go to waste. You can also choose a treatment moisturizer with a higher concentration of active ingredients that will go to work while you sleep.

7. Apply EYE CREAM.

Follow the directions for daytime.

EXFOLIATE EVERY WEEK

Did you know that Nefertiti was a big fan of exfoliation back in 1372 B.C., give or take a few years? She made sure to wash herself every morning with a mixture of water and natural lime water, rubbing her body with a clay paste made from Nile mud, and rubbing away rough spots on her body with pumice. She often followed that exfoliation with richly hydrating and soothing masks made from ostrich eggs, clay, oils, and milk. She couldn't have known the specific science behind why this system worked—only that it did. Because she was using natural exfoliants.

Fortunately, we don't need to crack open ostrich eggs anymore to improve our skin. Exfoliation is a very simple process, and yet I've found that many of the women I've talked to don't really understand what it actually is or how important it is for your beauty routine. It's by far the most effective way to wake up and improve a sluggish complexion.

The primary reason to exfoliate is because skin cells are very short-lived. They're formed, they migrate to the surface of your epidermis to form your stratum corneum, and they die. Teenagers and women in their twenties regenerate new skin cells about every twenty-eight to thirty days, but as you get older, this process can take more than fifty days. If you don't slough off these dead cells, they quickly start to accumulate—and this is what makes your complexion dull and your pores look larger.

I think the reason so many women are skittish about exfoliation is because they might have tried scrubbing with irritating substances—like jagged ground apricot pits—when they had acne or other teenage skin problems. Or they erroneously thought scrubbing was just part of the cleansing process. This left them with skin that became even more red and irritated due to the damage caused by the rough scrubs and the stripping away of skin's protective natural oils.

The best exfoliants are gentle and nonirritating

yet still effective. Choose one according to your skin type. Combination or oily skin can use a gentle daily exfoliant in place of a cleanser, while those with dry or sensitive skin should look for a gentle buffing cream with a mechanical exfoliant like nonirritating jojoba beads.

CHOOSE THE RIGHT MOISTURIZER FOR YOUR SKIN TYPE AND SKINCARE NEEDS

No matter what your skincare issue, you can find a moisturizer in all price ranges to treat it. The best brands have different textures for different issues, such as a firming moisturizer for oily skin and one for dry skin, so explore all your options until you find a moisturizer that suits you.

However old you are or whatever your skin type, the first thing you must look for is a moisturizer that contains antioxidants.

The best antioxidant ingredients include polyphenols and vitamin E (tocopherol).

Even if you've never used a good antioxidant moisturizer before, it's never too late! Mere weeks after you start applying an effective cream, you will see an improvement in the texture and appearance of your skin. You can't undo years of damage from the sun or smoking, but you can still make noticeable changes.

Moisturizers can be one of or a combination of any of these three types:

1. Antiwrinkle Moisturizers
The mere thought of wrinkles terrifies many women because they are such a visible sign of aging. Over the centuries, women desper-

ate to keep their skin firm have tried countless food items and chemical potions and aromatic yet toxic elixirs. A perfect example was the fabled Lola Montez, whose book *The Arts of Beauty: Or, Secrets of a Lady's Toilet,* was published in New York in 1858. In it she claimed, among other morsels, that a layer of beef suet applied to the face would help conceal wrinkles.

Aren't you glad you live in the twenty-first century?

MOISTURIZERS FOR YOUR AGE

* When you are in your twenties: Use an antioxidant moisturizer.

* When you are in your thirties: Use an antioxidant, antiwrinkle moisturizer.

* When you are in your forties: Use an antioxidant, antiwrinkle moisturizer that is also firming, as this is when skin starts to sag.

* When you are in your fifties and beyond: Use a moisturizer that is an all-in-one; it should contain antioxidants and be antiwrinkle and firming, tackle dark spots, and even out your skin tone. Some women are lucky enough to need only antioxidant moisturizers/brighteners because they have few, if any, wrinkles. This is true for many women of Asian descent because, as I explained in chapter 4, the extra fatty cells they have in their skin keep their skin plump and firm for longer.

One of the best skincare habits of the French is that we start using an antioxidant-laden antiwrinkle cream from a very early age. We know that this will keep our skin as hydrated and healthy as possible.

The best antiwrinkle ingredients include resveratrol, vitamin C, hyaluronic acid micro, peptides, and retinol.

2. Firming Moisturizers

Sagging and drooping skin is nearly as fearsome a thought as wrinkles. Ironically, women who are very thin, with extremely low levels of body fat, can actually seem to sag more than women their age who are a normal weight—that's because the fat pads underlying their facial muscles will disappear along with the fat everywhere else on their bodies, giving their skin less support. In addition, skin naturally loses firmness with age as collagen and elastin levels decline. You can combat this with a firming moisturizer. These work especially well if you have a V-shaped face, with a wider forehead than chin, which tends to make sagging more pronounced.

The best firming ingredients include resveratrol and firming peptides.

3. Brightening/Lightening/Evening Out Skin Tone/Hyperpigmentation Moisturizers

When we launched our Vinoperfect Radiance Serum in 2005, which is designed to brighten skin, it was not an immediate hit. Women just didn't know how to use it, or misunderstood what it was intended to do—which is to brighten, lighten, even out and improve your complexion, and give your skin a lovely glow.

Luckily, two French journalists turned the tables completely. One was a very heavy smoker, so her skin looked ashy all the time;

once she started using the serum twice a day, her complexion turned rosier and she looked a lot healthier. Did she stop smoking? No, even though she should have, of course. But when she wrote about our serum, legions of Frenchwomen who smoked ran out to get it. The other journalist brought the serum to Saint-Tropez when she was on vacation. She applied it underneath her sunscreen, and then wrote that her suntan lasted longer and she didn't get any freckles or splotches. That's all it took for the serum to become one of our top sellers. It still is, after all these years, in large part because it is the only serum on the market that can be used under sunscreen without losing any effectiveness, and even the most sensitive skins can use it without fear of irritation.

Hyperpigmentation sounds like a mouthful, but it's just a long word for an incredibly common condition, where tiny deposits of increased pigment appear on your skin, usually in the form of brownish spots or splotches.

Your skin contains cells called melanocytes; they produce melanin, the pigment that gives skin its coloration. The amount of melanin you have is genetically determined. Freckles appear when your melanocytes are damaged, usually on your face and limbs. Larger freckles, also known as age spots or liver spots, usually appear on your hands, chest, shoulders, arms, and upper back, especially on light-skinned people. As melanocytes are destroyed over time, white spots can also appear on your hands, arms, and legs. This is called melanosis, and it's the kind of sun damage that can't be undone.

Actually, I don't think these large freckles should be called *age* spots when they're almost always *sun-damage* spots. That's because the number one cause of hyperpigmentation is exposure to UV radiation.

Other typical causes are hormonal changes, such as birth control pills, pregnancy, or menopause; skin injury; or acne scar in response to a rash or a pimple. These healed blemishes are called postinflammatory hyperpigmentation and are often seen on women with darker skin tones. They can sometimes take a long time to go away, which is very frustrating.

The best brightening/hyperpigmentation ingredients include Viniferine, glycolic acid and papaya enzymes (to stimulate cell renewal), kojic acid, and bearberry extract. All these ingredients work only on abnormal pigmentation, so they are perfectly safe to use every day.

DON'T FORGET THE MASKS

A mask is a product with a higher concentration of active ingredients, designed to be left on your skin for a specific length of time and then rinsed off. I love masks and use them all the time. As you'll see in chapter 8, it's incredibly easy to make your own that are not only inexpensive but also highly effective. They are infinitely customizable, so you can create one for hydration, for soothing, for purifying, for detoxifying, for brightening, or just because it feels good. Also, if you apply a facial treatment oil with at least 5 percent essential oils underneath your mask, this will instantly boost its effectiveness.

TAKE GOOD CARE OF YOUR NECK!

The late writer and film director Nora Ephron wrote a hilarious book of essays I love called *I Feel Bad About My Neck*—and we can all sympathize! That's because the skin on your neck has fewer sebaceous glands, making it more delicate as well as slower to heal and repair itself, especially after a sunburn. It's also why women start seeing what they often call "chicken skin" long before the skin on their face is as wrinkled or loose. Once your neck skin has this kind of crepey texture, it becomes hard to treat (and you'll need to see a dermatologist about options, such as peels or lasers).

Like your lips—which are easy to neglect until they become chapped—you should always treat your neck as you treat your face. Don't stop at your chin—stop at your shoulders! Never forget sunscreen, which will help prevent crepiness from forming in the first place.

You don't need a specific product for your neck skin, but be sure to use a serum and a rich moisturizer or an antioxidant cream loaded with active ingredients. Even if your face is normal or oily, your neck skin is much more likely to be dry and dehydrated.

MY SKINCARE ROUTINE

The key for me is keeping it simple, with an emphasis on the best skincare rather than makeup. Without a great canvas, it's very difficult for makeup to be all that effective anyway. I have normal skin, and this is how I take care of my face:

- Cleansing. I use a foaming cleanser in the morning that is gentle and rinses off easily. At night, I use a cleansing oil.

- Beauty Elixir or Toner. The Caudalie Beauty Elixir is antibacterial, refreshes, and smoothes skin and minimizes pores. The Caudalie Moisturizing Toner adds more hydration to my skin and preps it for my serum and moisturizer.

- Serum. Depending on the season and how my skin feels, my serum will be hydrating, detoxifying, brightening, or firming.

- Moisturizers. For daytime, I apply one depending on whether or not I look tired. Usually, I use Vinoperfect tinted moisturizer with an SPF on top of my regular global anti-aging moisturizer (Premier Cru). For night, I use a moisturizer with glycolic acid to boost cell renewal and brighten, lighten, and even my skin, as it has a tendency to get dull, especially when I'm traveling.

- Eye Cream. I apply it all the way around my eye with my ring finger—and also around my lips, as it is extra-gentle and hydrating, and I like the texture better than that of a lip balm.

- Exfoliation. I exfoliate once a week with a mixture of jojoba microbeads, honey, and grape-seed oil, blending it with a foaming cleanser on my Clarisonic brush.

- Protecting my skin from free radicals and from the sun. Most of the time, in the gray sky of Paris, when I know I'll be spending the day inside, my tinted moisturizer with SPF 20 gives me the protection I need. If it's summer and I know I'll be outside in the sun a lot, I'll apply an SPF 50. But when I travel, the only moisturizer I bring with me is my all-in-one, one-and-done Premier Cru cream.

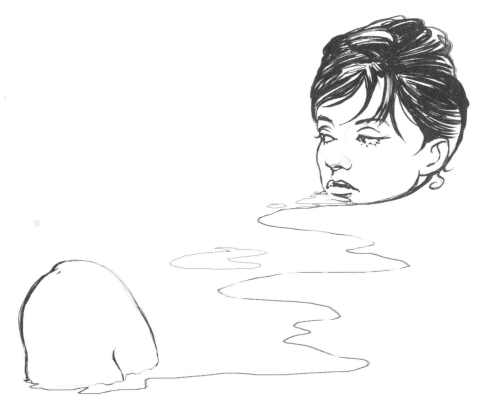

Seven

TAKING CARE OF YOUR BODY—
AND DON'T FORGET THE PERFUME!

For the French, skincare doesn't stop at the chin. Our *pharmacies* are loaded with wonderful products for all parts of the body—and we use them regularly. When you eat well and take care of yourself so that your figure is trim and slim, it's equally important to have skin that's not only glowing with health, but also properly hydrated, soft, and vibrant. Here's how.

THE ESSENCE OF FRENCH BODY CARE
YOU DON'T NEED LONG SHOWERS

Squeaky clean, as you know by now, is bad news for skin—often leaving it parched and flaky. Because much of the climate in France has historically been more moderate than in America, many homes were never equipped with effective central heating, and it often took quite a while for the water to get hot (and stay hot!). As a result, many Frenchwomen never got into the habit of taking long, steamy showers. When my sister and I would get ready for our showers, my grandmother used to tell us, "Don't soap all your body every day, just the part that smells!"

Decades later, I can see the wisdom in this. Hot water can feel wonderfully soothing, especially in cold weather or after a hard workout, but it's extremely drying. One of the best ways to counteract this is to turn off your shower and apply an oil all over your body—not just your arms and legs—*before* you towel off. A good oil, such as grape seed, argan, sweet almond, jojoba, or coconut, will soak right in, and the heat of the shower will have opened your pores, making them more receptive to any active ingredients in your moisturizing product. Then gently pat yourself dry.

In winter months when the frigid air and super-dry heating leave your skin even drier, you can apply another light layer of a hydrating cream or oil when you're totally dry. Think of this technique as a moisture sandwich for your skin. It really needs to be an essential part of your daily routine, because skin can get so dry so quickly, and the last thing you want when you're bundled up against the cold is itchy, flaky skin.

Don't forget to pay particular attention to your elbows and ears, as they are often neglected. Your ears, in particular, can get terribly sun damaged over the years, because it's so easy to forget to put sunscreen on them. This is, scarily enough, one of the reasons why ears are a prime location for skin cancers.

Speaking of ears, Régine, Caudalie's lead esthetician and trainer at the Caudalie Spa in New York City, has told me that she now sees a lot of clients with blackheads and other spots on their ears due to cell phone use. They used to appear on our chins back in the days when all we had in the office were landlines and heavy handsets that we'd cradle on our faces all day—at least those spots are long gone!

Finally, if you want an instant energy boost, try finishing your bath or shower with a blast of cold water, which tones and firms the skin by enhancing microcirculation.

French Beauty Secret

For an anytime scrub, simply mix one tablespoon of baking soda with water until you have a paste. Rub it gently on, then rinse with warm water. This is an instant way to get rid of dead skin cells and give your skin that special glow.

HIGH ON THE LIST OF THINGS THAT GIVE FRENCHWOMEN NIGHTMARES IS CELLULITE

My mother is the envy of all her friends. Not just because she is my wonderful and adored *maman* or because her wine is so delicious. They envy her because she has absolutely no cellulite. When you look at her from behind she has the smooth and taut legs and bottom of a sixteen-year-old. I think her secret is that she religiously massages the areas of the body where cellulite can show up. And when I say religiously, that is an understatement! She also frequently visits the Caudalie Spa on her vineyard and trains the high-powered jets of water in the treatment rooms on her skin to help with circulation, just in case—but even if she'd never set foot in a spa, she'd still have no cellulite!

My mother is not unique in her fight against these annoying

dimples. Teenagers in other countries might be obsessed with makeup or boy bands or dating, but in France they're obsessed with cellulite. Cellulite is caused by fat cells that get trapped in your body's connective tissue, close to the surface of the skin; this is why it's so visible, and why liposuction, which is designed to remove fat found in deeper skin layers, can paradoxically make cellulite worse.

Never mind that there is a huge genetic component to cellulite as well—which is why women who are slim, toned, and fit can still have it (just take a look at tennis players for a perfect example; they're world-class athletes in prime condition and can still have cellulite). Losing weight can slightly reduce cellulite, but plenty of women who've always been slender still have it. Never mind that there is still no cure for it or any treatment that is guaranteed to be permanently effective. Whoever can invent a truly permanent process to get rid of cellulite would have the undying gratitude of millions of women.

Topical treatments such as creams that you rub on or professional treatments, including the Frenchwoman's favorite, *endermologie cellu M6*, which is a deep-tissue massage-type machine, can make a visible difference in cellulite's appearance—but regular sessions are needed and the results aren't permanent. Frenchwomen are much more avid consumers of slimming creams and contouring creams than American women tend to be. It's not that we believe we're going to lose five pounds if we rub on a cream, but we do know that the massaging we do when we apply the product makes it work better. For the professional massages done at the Caudalie Spa in Bordeaux, I used a combination of essential oils of lemon, lemongrass, juniper, cypress, rosemary, and geranium in a base of grape-seed oil, followed by a high-dosage caffeine cream, and I've found that this combination has a noticeable effect.

(This formula is now in Caudalie's Contouring Concentrate.) Most over-the-counter skincare products for use on your legs that claim to specifically target cellulite (they're often called "slimming" or "contouring" creams) contain caffeine, as it has an immediate, though temporary, tightening effect.

The reason massage works so well is due to your body's lymphatic system, which helps remove waste. Massaging certain points of the body helps get sluggish lymph fluid moving better, removing toxins. I love using a little roller for self-massage and keep it handy all the time—even when I'm driving (at least I'm being productive when stuck in traffic!). Usually, though, I use a massage oil with a stimulating effect, like the one I just mentioned, every day. I apply it to damp skin after my shower and massage it in using circular movements. Start at your feet and move upward, concentrating on any problem areas. Using a small device like a hand roller makes the massage more effective.

REGULAR EXFOLIATION KEEPS SKIN GLOWING

Just as you need to exfoliate your facial skin, so should you exfoliate your body at least once a week. This will keep your skin looking fresh and smooth. It's incredibly easy to do this in the shower or bath.

Exfoliating scrubs usually have a base of either sugars or salts. I prefer sugars, as salts can sting if you have little cuts or blisters. One of Caudalie's bestselling products is our Crushed Cabernet Scrub with a brown sugar base, and the recipe on page 198 in the next chapter will show you how to make it at home. They are great for use in a bath, but in a regular scrub you want something that's not as abrasive and won't pull out moisture from your skin. Sugar bonds with water, which makes it hydrating as well as an effective exfoliant.

IS THERE ANY WAY TO GET RID OF STRETCH MARKS?

Stretch marks are a bit like cellulite, as your body's tendency to have them is genetic, and they are, unfortunately, permanent. I know women who have always been thin, but once they hit puberty and started growing, stretch marks appeared on their hips (much to their frustration!). They can also appear during periods of rapid weight gain, such as pregnancy or yo-yo dieting. If you do have them, speak to your dermatologist. Stretch marks are easier to treat with topical products when they're new and still red. Once they turn white, lasers are one of the only options and they aren't always successful. If you do see them during pregnancy, the best thing you can do is keep your skin as moisturized as possible. Otherwise, keeping your weight stable is the best preventative measure you can take.

HANDS NEED SPECIAL CARE

Like the skin under your eyes, the skin on your hands is thinner and more transparent than skin found on the rest of your body. Frenchwomen are well aware of this, which is one of the reasons Caudalie's hand cream is one of our bestselling products in France. We also know what damage can be done by the regular use of hand sanitizers. These gels are fantastic for keeping germs at bay and surfaces clean, but most of them are composed primarily of alcohol, which is extremely drying. Always apply a good hand cream after your hand sanitizer—keep the containers next to each other or stashed in a little bag in your purse so it's easy to remember. Keep a container on your nightstand and apply a thick layer of a rich cream before bed, too.

Be sure to test hand creams before you purchase them. The cream should feel luxurious but should absorb right away without leaving an oily residue—it should feel like a protective little glove. As you know from chapter 5, you should avoid products with mineral oil as one of the top ingredients, as it's unctuous and can clog your pores. Instead, look for creams containing powerful antioxidants and nourishing ingredients like plant oils.

And because hand skin is so delicate and exposed to the elements, it often shows signs of photoaging long before your face or arms. I like to rub the excess sunscreen from my face onto my

French Beauty Secret

One of the easiest ways to keep your hands looking young is by cultivating a glove collection and wearing them regularly. Frenchwomen adore gloves in brightly colored leathers or fabrics and change up their pairs the way they change up their sunglasses— they're a great addition to your accessories collection. Don't just think of gloves as something to keep your hands warm in winter. You can even wear lightweight cotton gloves in the summer, which is an ideal way to prevent sun damage.

hands every morning so I don't forget to put it on. If you start to see brown hyperpigmentation spots, use a brightening product like any of those mentioned in chapter 6 and always follow with a high-SPF sunscreen.

Hands can also be exfoliated when you're doing the rest of your body. Consider them part of your French face—but use a very gentle exfoliant to mitigate irritation.

NAILS NEED LOVE, TOO

I'll never understand how the French manicure got its name because I've never seen one in Paris.

But the French do take care of their nails. Like your hair, your nails are composed of dead protein, and they can get very dry and brittle, especially during winter months or in rooms with low humidity. Toenails often suffer from extreme dryness, especially when you're wearing closed shoes. If you like to get frequent manicures, the chemicals in the polish remover as well as in the polish itself can be drying and irritating. Fake nails are also chemical-based and can damage the nail bed, so I would not recommend their use. Frenchwomen tend to keep their nails very short and low-maintenance, with either unobtrusive neutrals or classic red if we use any polish, although we are beginning to follow the American lead a bit more and get more adventurous with our colors, particularly on our toes.

There are a few simple rules for nail care, whether on your hands or feet:

- If the edges of your nails are starting to peel, that means your nails are super-dry and need extra hydration. Use an emollient product like jojoba, avocado, neem, or apricot oil, and soak your nails in it for a few minutes, or massage in a few drops.

Try doing so after your bath or shower, as your cuticles will be very soft, and you can push them back with a towel and then apply the oil. Or try adding a few drops of essential oil of geranium or lemon to grape-seed oil, as this will fortify your nails. You really can't overdo this moisturization of your nails, and any excess oil or cream will be soaked up by your fingers, leaving them soft, too.

- Never cut your cuticles, as that can lead to infections. Simply apply a natural source of hydration like neem or apricot oil, rub it in well, and push them back with your fingers or a towel after every bath or shower. Eventually, they'll stay in place. Avoid the cuticle sticks nail salons often use, as they aren't hygienic and can easily tear your cuticles. If you like to use them at home, wrap some soft cotton around the pointed end to be gentler on your nails.

- Use a nail hardener. I love Herôme, which I've found is the very best product for stronger nails, and all my friends use it, too. It's easy to find it online.

- Consider taking a supplement to help with nail growth. I like the brand Phyto, available online.

French Beauty Secret

Keep your nail polish in the fridge. It will last a lot longer and go on more smoothly.

KEEP YOUR FEET SOFT

As with hand cream, Frenchwomen are avid buyers of foot cream. There are twenty-four thousand *pharmacies* in France (one for every five thousand people). I love walking into them, and I've yet to see a *pharmacie* anywhere in France that doesn't have a prominently displayed foot-cream section. American drugstores, on the other hand, rarely highlight their footcare products—they're often positioned on the lower shelves, too, making them hard to find. This is a shame, because a little bit of footcare reaps great rewards. No one wants to have cracked heels or brittle toenails, and it's very simple to remedy this with daily use of a foot cream.

Look for a product that contains nourishing plants and oils like shea butter, grape-seed oil, and glycerin, as well as red vine lead and ginkgo to improve circulation. Like hand cream, the product should not be greasy and it should absorb instantly so you don't worry about slipping when you walk or about staining your sheets. Apply this cream right before bed and then put your hand cream on afterward.

French Beauty Secret

Sleep with lightweight cotton socks on after you slather on your foot cream. It will help your cream absorb better (and not get all over your sheets or be slippery when you walk). It may not be sexy, but once you start doing this your feet will be much smoother and you won't need to do it every night.

BEAUTY ON THE GO

I love the adventures I can have on the road, whether for business or pleasure. But I don't love going to airports and standing in endless lines, often with plans upended due to weather or other delays. And then there is the circulating air on the planes to deal with. The average humidity level during a flight hovers around 10 percent, which is drier than a desert! I needed to develop a travel routine that keeps my skin in top condition no matter where I'm going.

- Moisturize your face as well as your entire body before getting on the plane. Really slather it on. In fact, you can use a thin layer of a moisturizing mask instead of your regular cream and keep it on during your entire flight. Don't forget your lips and hands—use a thick cream on your hands and reapply often.

- Once you get in your seat, change the time on your watch to the time at your destination as you board your flight. This mental trick helps you adjust and minimizes jet lag.

- I never leave home without my earplugs and sleeping mask.

- Try not to eat while flying, if possible. I know this is tough, especially if you have a long flight, but airplane food tends to be very un-healthy, and is often overloaded with sodium and other preservatives that can cause you to store water and become very bloated. (Not to mention that excessive sodium levels are terri-ble for heart health, as they raise your blood pressure.) If your flight is very long and you know you'll get hungry, bring food such as ap-ples and bananas, if possible, as they are satiat-ing and easy to digest.

- Drink plenty of water. Then drink more! As much as I try to avoid bottled water, this is the one time where bringing a large bottle with me is a must. Stay away from anything carbon-ated, as it can leave you extra-bloated.

- One glass of red wine at most. I know that it is far more potent at altitude and extremely de-hydrating. Still, I love my nightly glass of red wine, so I have one small glass, especially if it's a night flight, as it helps me to sleep.

THE FRENCH LOVE AFFAIR WITH PERFUME

What could be more French than French perfume? For women around the world, a bottle of Chanel No. 5 or Shalimar is the height of sophistication.

The French have the Italian Catherine de Medici, wife of King Henri II, to thank for bringing the Renaissance Italian perfume techniques to the French court in the 1530s. Catherine adored her perfumer, Rene the Florentine, so much that she had a secret passageway built in the palace so no one could inhale any of the preciously guarded formulas before she did. In 1656, Maître Parfumeur et Gantier (Master Glover of Perfumes), the guild of glove and perfume making was formed, and scented gloves became all the rage. These gloves continued to be extremely popular during the reigns of Louis XIV and Louis XV, as the glove makers figured out a way to infuse the leather with different scents during the tanning process. (An homage to these techniques can be found at the MPG boutique on rue des Capucines in Paris now, where you can still purchase scented gloves and many different perfumes.)

Louis XIV was partial to iris root and scented not only his skin—giving him the nickname Le Doux Fleurant, or the Sweet-Smelling—but also his clothing, wigs, handkerchiefs, fans, furniture, and fountains. During his reign, more than three hundred *parfumeries* opened in Paris, and they quickly became the go-to salons for aristocrats. His son Louis XV loved perfume just as much if not more, so much so that during his reign Versailles was nicknamed *la cour parfumée* (the perfumed court). After the Revolution, Napoleon managed to go through two quarts of violet cologne every week and sixty bottles of jasmine every month, while his wife, Josephine, drenched herself in so much musk that her rooms remained scented for decades thereafter!

Thanks to the patronage of the courtiers, the perfume industry flourished, in large part due to the climate of the south of France, particularly in Grasse. This town was ideal for growing jasmine, rose, lavender, mimosa, and oranges, and it became the principal supplier for perfumers based in Paris—a tradition that continues today.

I have always loved scent, as you know, and from a young age I wanted to work in the fragrance business. I would go into Grenoble and spend hours smelling the different scents in the local *parfumeries*—they fascinated me and I memorized dozens of them. When my mother's friends came over, they were astonished because I could recognize their perfume, which was usually Guerlain's L'Heure Bleue, and worried they'd put too much on. My father was very impressed and encouraged me to do an internship in fragrance, and I was able to do my first one at Cacharel when I was only about fifteen. It was amazing training being around all those incredible noses, who are true artists of scent, and scent has always been an extremely important part of all Caudalie products. When a cream or a cleanser smells wonderful, not only does it make you much more likely to use it, but it's also going to make you feel good, too.

French Beauty Secret

Take a tip from chic Parisians and spray a cotton handkerchief with your favorite fragrance and keep it in your handbag. Everything will smell divine each time you open your bag. You can also place a scented handkerchief inside your leather gloves to scent them as well. And take another tip from Marilyn Monroe, who famously kept her Chanel No. 5 in the fridge in *The Seven Year Itch*. Perfume should never be stored in a bathroom or on a shelf near a window, as heat and humidity affect the potency of the scent.

WHAT INSPIRES ME

The natural world has always been one of my most profound inspirations, and what I especially love is to match the best of what nature has to offer with the most innovative modern techniques.

To live in harmony with the natural world has always been my family's philosophy. When my parents moved to Château Smith Haut Lafitte, the vines were overrun and the fields fallow, and they decided that they would bring the vineyard back to life by natural means. That meant biodiversity; organic compost; natural pheromones to banish moths and mites and prevent the grapes from rot; and flowers planted to entice the bees and other pollinating insects. We harvest every single grape by hand. You can't get more natural than that.

When I need to recharge, all my senses are inspired, soothed, and made joyous by this vineyard. Nothing is more wonderful than the sweet, pungent scents: the delicate perfume of the grape blossoms, the intoxicating woody scent in the cooperage where we make the barrels from freshly cut French oak and roast the oak to prime it for the wine, the enveloping softness of the orangery, the green crispness as the wind blows through the cypress trees, the aroma of the Earl Grey tea that we sip at the end of the day as the sky begins to darken.

But no matter where I am, my environment constantly inspires me. I am constantly amazed and in-spired by the noise and the energy and the lights and the boundless enthusiasm I find in New York City. I like starting my day like a cannonball. No lingering in a French café when there's work to be done, *bien sur!*

Even though I left my path toward a career in the perfume industry, scent has always been extremely important to me. Especially the marvelous scents from the beverages I like to drink: lime tea, fresh mint, melissa from the garden, pungent Rooibos tea from South Africa, all the notes from different grape varieties—the white peach and citrus fruits from the Sauvignon Blanc, the sweet and spicy notes from the Cabernet, the fullness of the red berries from the Merlot.

I'm also inspired all the time by my research and development team. I'm passionate about my work, and I'm constantly testing—sometimes up to a hundred times until the formulas are truly fin-ished. No matter what their endeavor, I find the dedication of people striving to do their very best to be incredibly inspirational. It keeps me on my toes and it expands my own thinking, too.

HOW TO FIND YOUR SIGNATURE SCENT

One of my favorite scents when I was about twelve was grapefruit. That summer, my mother went to Roland Garros stadium for a French tennis tournament, and she came back with a bottle of perfume called Double Mix, made for that tournament. It had a heavy citrus base, and I was crazy about the tangy grapefruit notes. My mother gave me the bottle because, at the time, she was devoted to Cinnabar from Estée Lauder, which as you can imagine from the name was heavy on the spicy side. I always knew when she was home because I could smell her before I saw her. This drove my grandmother crazy because she liked only old-fashioned, super-light florals, which were the antithesis of Cinnabar. It took years for my mother to find a different signature scent.

I didn't mind it, though. Nearly every woman I know has happy memories of themselves as little girls, watching *maman* at her *toilette*, getting ready for the night and spraying on a delicious perfume before going out to dinner or a party; how grown-up and seductive it was!

Some of my friends or colleagues will stick to one signature scent, thrilled that they've found one that perfectly suits their personality. That makes me happy, as I always know who it is before she even walks in the room, and it can also conjure up scent memories of, perhaps, the first time you smelled it on her and what you were doing at the time (even if that time was many years ago!). Others joyfully refer to themselves as perfume junkies and have an endlessly growing scent wardrobe, which they use as an accessory to match their mood, or their outfit, or just because the scent pleases them that day. Scent is such an idiosyncratic thing that there's no right or wrong to it—unless you're wearing too much of an overpowering fragrance. The most important thing to remember is to have fun with fragrance and play around with it as you do your fashion or makeup. Think of it as one of the most potent accessories in your closet—as interchangeable as a pair of sunglasses or high heels. Perfume is one of the easiest ways to make yourself unique—because no "true" fragrance smells exactly the same from one person to another.

You should also trust your senses. It's hard to put words to a scent, particularly if you're not sure what the notes in it are, so you need to close your eyes and rely solely on your nose to see if you like it or not. The bottle might look incredible but it's only what's inside that counts, so ignore the packaging. Some of the most amazing fragrances I've ever smelled are created by noses, especially the independent brands I love, who care more about the juice than the bottles, and the only way to know is to try one on.

I would also advise you not to ever buy a perfume when you first smell it, as a good perfume has several layers: The top note is what you first smell; the middle develops after a minute or two; and the base or bottom note is the truest aspect of the perfume and the one that will linger. (If you become seriously interested in perfume, the websites www.basenotes.net or www.osmoz.com break down hundreds of different perfumes into their top, middle, and base so you can better understand what's in the scent.) Depending on your unique chemistry, a perfume can undergo an amazing transformation as it deepens, and you might find yourself loving (or loathing) something that smelled completely different at first whiff. Or, sometimes you can be wildly disappointed when a friend discovers something that smells absolutely incredible on her but it just doesn't work on you. That's why it's essential to try perfume on your skin and avoid the testing sticks, as it's the only way to get an accurate result. Scent is like clothing—it might look great on the hanger, but when you try it on, it either enhances your figure or just doesn't work. You won't know till you try.

For me, perfume is like music you wear. It can grate (if it's the wrong kind of tune or the wrong kind of scent for you) or make you incredibly happy and uplifted (when the music soars to match your mood and the perfume just smells so incredibly good). Be adventurous and have fun! Test and test until you find just the right scent for you—many stores are happy to give you samples. Just be sure not to test too many at once, as it will be hard to differentiate between them, and you need to let the fragrance develop its true nature over time, as you know. Test no more than two— one on each wrist—at a time, and be sure to remember which is which. (If you want to test more, what better excuse do you need to go back to the store and sample something else!) Invite your friends over for a perfume party, and sample each other's favorites. Change your perfume with the seasons; what smells bright and fresh in summer heat might be too light for cold and dark days of winter, when you want a potent scent that is darker and more complicated.

There are thousands of amazing fragrances made by talented noses around the world. The website LuckyScent features many of these most unique and daring boutique perfumes. They can be very expensive, but this site allows you to buy small samples at small prices, so you can properly test a perfume that you'd never know about otherwise. Who knows—you might just fall in love!

HOW I CREATED ROSE DE VIGNE

My personal preference is for fragrances that are very natural, as you know, and all the Caudalie fragrances are inspired by the many intoxicating scents of the vineyard. For example, Zeste de Vigne is based on the winter garden at the *château*, where the orange, mandarin, and lemon trees are in bloom and the deeply scented neroli and petitgrain perfumes the air, in contrast to the chill and wind outside. Figue de Vigne is very summery, fruity and bright; Thé des Vignes has musky overtones, inspired by all the scents wafting in a breeze at sunset; and Fleur de Vigne is a fresh floral that reminds you of the springtime blossoms of the vine flowers.

For Rose de Vigne I had in my mind the lovely yellow rose that's planted on the edge of every single grapevine row in my parents' vineyard, because if the fragile roses start to show any sign of disease, you know to treat the grapes. Not only do these roses smell divine, but they are also natural guardian angels for the precious grapes—isn't that amazing? I wanted to capture the scent of the rose as it smells early in the morning, with the dew still on the petals, mingling with the fresh, green, earthy scent of the dew-laden grapevines and the chlorophyll of the bright green leaves.

I wanted a complex, modern, green kind of rose-based scent, not one that was fusty or one-note, and I also wanted to cut the sweetness and prettiness of the rose with the crisp astringency of rhubarb, which I absolutely adore. The idea was to create a perfume that was airy, crisp, feminine, and sensual. Countless versions were tested over many months until it was right, with a top note of rose and rhubarb, middle notes of magnolia and lily of the valley, and a base of musk and amber.

French Beauty Secret

Your nose literally gets tired after inhaling just a few new scents and will be unable to tell them apart. A nifty trick is to deeply inhale the scent of fresh coffee beans in between sniffs. For some reason, this "resets" your nose and allows you to start testing again. This is why you'll often see little glasses of coffee beans on the counters in *parfumeries* all over the world.

Because my friends know that I'm not so much of a rose-fragrance lover, it's been a lot of fun to see how they react when they don't know I've sprayed it on. Often I hear, "Yum, you smell good, you smell fresh, what is it?" And I am always thrilled to tell them.

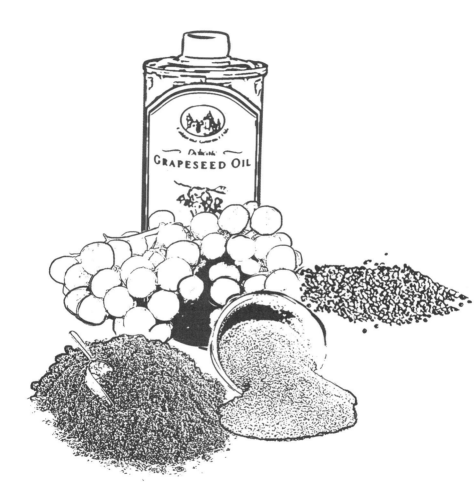

Eight

MY FAVORITE RECIPES

Customizing your skincare regimen is incredibly easy and inexpensive, especially with homemade masks. Use these regularly, as your skin will soak them up and always look better afterward.

Many of the masks include plain, unsweetened, full-fat yogurt. It's a terrific food for your skin as it contains lactic acid that is a gentle exfoliant, pore-shrinker, and moisturizer. Honey is also often used, as it naturally has antibiotic, antiviral, soothing, and hydrating properties—plus it smells divine. I use honey a lot in my products because it can speed healing and prevent infection. It also keeps moisture close to the skin, which can help your complexion become supple and glowing.

This chapter offers natural DIY recipes to help augment whatever you buy at the store. It's organized based on your skin type and problem you're trying to solve. I love homemade recipes because they're a great way to try lots of different products without breaking the bank or committing to something before you know it works. Those you'll find here are the best of my favorites from my family as well as from Caudalie's therapists in France and around the world.

Note: Whatever the ingredient, it's very important that it be of the highest possible quality. Use organic fruits and vegetables, cold-pressed organic oils, raw honey, and organic milk. The recipes won't be as effective if you don't use the best—and you certainly don't want to put the residue of any pesticides or other chemicals on your skin from nonorganic products.

French Beauty Secret

One of the easiest ways to decongest and hydrate your skin is with a cucumber. Make sure the cucumber is cold (it needs to have been refrigerated for at least twenty minutes). Slice it thinly, lie down, and apply slices all over your face. Remove after ten minutes.

IF YOU HAVE DRY OR DEHYDRATED SKIN

When your skin is dry or dehydrated, you need extra pampering and vigilant care to keep it smooth and hydrated. You should use a serum every day and a rich cream at night when it can penetrate your skin and the active ingredients can get to work. Go for creamy cleansers that you remove with a gentle toner. Try to avoid using hot water to wash your face, as it's very drying. In addition, masks are ideal for adding extra moisture, so get into the habit of using them regularly.

SERUM

I love to customize my serums, and all you have to do is add a drop or two of essential oil to any serum of your choice for its therapeutic properties. You can also try using a hydrating serum in the morning and a detoxifying serum at night, which will help de-stress your skin from the daily assaults made on it.

When Les Sources de Caudalie Vinotherapie Spa in Bordeaux opened in 1999, my estheticians asked me to create serums with a blend of different essential oils, as I knew which oils would work well together and be especially effective for specific conditions our clients might have. You can easily do the same at home. There are many reputable websites of herbalists that sell essential oils, bottles, and other supplies, and most of the oils are inexpensive and last for a very long time. You'll also find essential oils at health-food stores and some drugstores.

Use a small, dark glass bottle with a stopper for each potion and be sure to label it. Fill it 95 percent full of the plant-based oil or oils of your choice, and then add a few drops of different essential oils. (The essential oils should be no more than 5 percent of the potion.) Mix and match as you like. Store them away from heat and light.

Use six drops of these potions in place of your regular serum at night. In addition, you can apply a few drops under your moisturizer, add up to twenty drops to your bath, or blend a few drops into your body lotion.

For moisturizing

Base oils: Grape seed, hazelnut, jojoba oil, almond, muskrose.
Essential oils: Rose, palmarosa.

For detox

Base oils: Grape seed, musk rose, sweet almond.

Essential oils: Lavender, bitter orange leaf, neroli, carrot seed, sandalwood.

For balancing

Base oils: Grape seed, jojoba.

Essential oils: Carrot, catnip, eucalyptus, lemon, lemongrass, melissa.

For slimming/cellulite (use on your body only)

Base oil: Grape seed.

Essential oils: Lemongrass, lemon, juniper berries, cypress, rosemary, geranium.

ANTIOXIDANT/ANTIWRINKLE TREATMENTS

In addition to your daily product, use this mask once a week.

Antioxidant Tomato Mask

1 medium tomato, smashed with a fork

1 teaspoon honey

1 teaspoon milk

1 teaspoon flour

- Mix all the ingredients together.
- Apply to face.
- Leave on for 15 minutes.
- Rinse with warm water.

BRIGHTENING/HYPERPIGMENTATION

In addition to your daily product, use this mask once a week.

Brightening and Soothing Mask

A few strawberries, smashed with a fork and mixed until smooth
$\frac{1}{3}$ to $\frac{1}{2}$ cup plain yogurt

- Mix strawberries and yogurt.
- Apply to your entire face.
- Leave on for 15 minutes.
- Rinse with warm water.

EXFOLIATION

As you know, once a week I'll add a bit of my cleansing mixture to a deep exfoliating scrub. You can use either of these masks once or twice a week.

Vitamin E Yogurt Mask

2 or 3 vitamin E capsules
$\frac{1}{3}$ to $\frac{1}{2}$ cup plain yogurt

- Empty the capsules into the yogurt and stir well.
- Apply to your entire face.
- Leave on for 10 to 15 minutes.
- Rinse with warm water.

Avocado Honey Yogurt Mask

½ avocado, pit removed

1 teaspoon honey

4 ounces plain yogurt

- Mix all ingredients well.
- Apply to your entire face.
- Leave on for 20 minutes.
- Rinse with warm water.

*This can also be used as a hair mask—it'll leave your hair super-shiny.

IF YOU HAVE NORMAL SKIN

Lucky you! You can use just about any product, so have fun experimenting. Just don't take your skin for granted, as you still need to wash it, exfoliate once a week, and hydrate, especially if the air in your home or office is dry.

BRIGHTENING/HYPERPIGMENTATION

This will give you instant radiance and is super-simple: Mix 1 teaspoon of instant oatmeal with enough water to make a paste. Gently rub it all over your face and rinse off. It's also suitable for all skin types.

EXFOLIATION

This scrub is great for dry skin, too.

Normal/Dry Skin Scrub

½ teaspoon regular (not instant) oatmeal
⅓ teaspoon sugar
1 tablespoon olive oil

- Mix all ingredients together.
- Rub gently on your face.
- Remove with tepid water and a washcloth.

MASKS

Use these masks, or choose any that you like from the other sections, especially if your skin is feeling a little dry or sluggish. Use them once a week.

Moisture Mask

This is ideal for all skin types.

3 tablespoons Greek yogurt
1 banana, mashed
1 teaspoon honey

- Mix all ingredients together.
- Let it dry for 20 minutes on your face.
- Rinse it off with warm water.

Detoxifying Mask

Because you don't need as many treatment products as other skin types, using this detoxifying mask is a terrific way to purify your skin from environmental aggressions, especially from pollution. It will erase imperfections and leave your skin soft and smooth. This mask can be used on all skin types, too.

1 teaspoon brewer's yeast
1 teaspoon milk
1 tablespoon honey
3 ounces plain yogurt
Rosewater (optional)

- Mix the yeast and milk together in a small glass bowl and place on a warm surface (like a radiator, the inside of a turned-off oven, or a shelf near a window on a sunny day) for 30 minutes. You should see bubbles in the milk.
- Whisk in the honey and yogurt.
- Let it dry for 10 minutes on your face.
- Rinse it off with warm water.
- Finish with a wipe of rosewater, which tightens your pores.

Honey and Lemon Mask

This mask has a dual purpose: moisturizing and exfoliating. The honey adds hydration while the enzymes in the lemon juice will help slough off dead skin cells.

¼ cup honey
1 tablespoon lemon juice

- Stir the honey and lemon juice together until smooth.
- Apply to your entire face.
- Leave on for 10 minutes.
- Rinse with warm water.

DIY SKINCARE SECRETS FROM THE FRENCH ARISTOCRACY

Going back centuries to when aristocrats ruled France, beauty has always held an important role in how Frenchwomen present themselves—whether to the courts, their kings, their husbands, or their lovers. They endlessly experimented with what was available to them at the time to keep their complexions glowing.

DIANE DE POITIERS, 1499–1556

Diane de Poitiers was the beloved mistress of King Henri II. Her glowing complexion was a result of her early-morning routine—she got up, had a cool bath, and then went for a long ride on horseback. Despite this healthy habit, though, when her remains were dug up several years ago (her tomb had been desecrated during the French Revolution and her body moved), forensic experts found mercury in her bones and high levels of gold in her hair. They theorized that she drank a potion of liquid gold in the mistaken belief that it would keep her skin looking young. She was very fortunate this potion didn't kill her at an early age.

MADAME DE POMPADOUR, 1721–1764

"Champagne is the only wine that leaves a woman beautiful after drinking it."

Adored mistress of King Louis XIV, Madame de Pompadour was never known as a great beauty—in fact, she was often described as quite plain. But her charm was so legendary that many considered her one of the loveliest women they'd ever met. How French is that! She also took immaculate care of her skin, applying lemon juice as a toner and then moisturizing with fresh carrot juice mixed with a teaspoon of honey, or sometimes with olive oil, and made a special mask of whipped cream and lemon juice (note how she was using fruit acids long before cosmetics companies did!).

MARIE ANTOINETTE, 1755–1793

Marie Antoinette loved her baths, especially when they were filled with detoxifying (and delicious) Champagne. She'd exfoliate with muslin pads infused with bran and used soaps compounded from herbs, bergamot, and amber. When her skin was looking dull, an egg white mask helped unclog her pores. She also wore gloves lined with wax, rosewater, and sweet almond oil every night—a precursor to the paraffin treatments often done in nail salons today. Back then, there were only two choices for face powder: ground-up white pearls, vinegar, and egg whites, which had a bit of a smell; or white chalk made from toxic lead, which over time could be lethal. And her blush was likely concocted from ground-up South American cochineal insects. At least *that* wasn't toxic.

EMPRESS JOSEPHINE, 1763–1814

Josephine grew up on the Caribbean island of Martinique and had learned many beauty tricks from the peasants who worked for her wealthy Creole family on their sugar plantation. She'd start the day with a glass of water mixed with a little bit of lemon juice and washed her face with camphor-infused compresses. She was also well-known for a face wash made from mixing fresh aloe vera gel with milk or cream—an ideal blend of an exfoliant (the acids in milk) with a moisturizer (the hydrating gel). You can easily try making this wash at home and see if it works for you, too.

IF YOU HAVE OILY OR COMBINATION NORMAL/OILY SKIN

When your skin is oily, your biggest issue is usually shine and imperfections such as pimples, blackheads, and enlarged pores. Look for ingredients that are purifying but not aggressive, especially if you have acne, as using harsh antibacterial creams or scrubs will often further inflame your skin. Oils are often great for cleansing, as they're soothing and moisturizing. At the top of my list are hazelnut and grape-seed oils, as they are slightly astringent and nongreasy.

Those with combination normal/oily skin tend to get shiny in some areas—often the T-zone—and are either normal or even a bit dry elsewhere, especially in winter. This can complicate your regimen when you want to dry up the shine without drying the areas that don't need it. You can use pretty much any cleanser that you like—but remember, the goal is never to be squeaky-clean or super-scrubbed. That strips all the good oils off your face and paradoxically makes your face produce even more of its own oil in compensation.

CLEANSER

To reduce excess oil, mix a few drops of grapefruit, sage, or cedar essential oils into your favorite cleanser.

SERUM

Make your own serum by mixing a few drops of lavender essential oil and tea tree oil or lemon, lemongrass, eucalyptus, balm mint, and melissa into a few tablespoons of jojoba or grape-seed oil. Keep it in a small glass jar with a dropper. Use it at night.

MOISTURIZER

If your skin is very oily, you might be able to forego this and just use an eye cream because that area always tends to be drier than the rest of your face.

BRIGHTENING/HYPERPIGMENTATION

You can follow any of the suggestions for other skin types.

EXFOLIATION
Scrub for Oily/Combination Skin

1 egg white
½ tablespoon regular (not instant) oatmeal
1 teaspoon lemon juice
⅓ teaspoon salt

- Mix all ingredients together.
- Rub gently on your face.
- Remove with tepid water and a washcloth.

Blackhead Remover

1 tablespoon baking soda
Water

- Mix baking soda and water to make a paste.
- Massage on your nose area for 30 seconds.
- Remove with tepid water and a washcloth.

MASKS

Look for astringent ingredients such as lemon, cucumber, honey, or yogurt—but only in small amounts. Your skin might be oily but it still needs soft and balancing ingredients like almond and jojoba oils, lavender essential oil, and rosewater.

Pore-Soothing Mask

1 egg white
1 tablespoon honey
1 tablespoon flour or cornstarch

- Whip the egg white with a fork until it's foamy.
- Slowly add the honey and flour or cornstarch.
- Leave it on your skin for 15 minutes.
- Remove with tepid water and a washcloth.

IF YOU HAVE SENSITIVE SKIN

If your skin is sensitive, the best thing to do is use as few products as needed, and with as few ingredients as possible. Your skin particularly needs calming and nonaggressive treatments. You should test every new product to see if you're allergic—simply apply a small dab on the inside of your arm and wait ten minutes to see if there is any kind of reaction.

MOISTURIZER

Fresh aloe vera gel is soothing enough for even the most sensitive skins. (It's also great for sunburns.) If you can find a piece of the aloe vera leaf, which is very thick, slice it open and rub the gel on your skin. You can also buy pure aloe vera gel at drugstores and health-food stores. This will also help tighten your pores while providing a lovely bit of hydration.

TONER

Avoid any toners that have alcohol as a base.

MASKS AND OTHER TREATMENTS

It's best not to concoct your own when your skin is sensitive. Stick to products that are hypoallergenic.

French Beauty Secret

Eye creams can be used around your lips, too. Or you can make your own lip exfoliant by mixing a very small amount of finely granulated brown sugar and honey together. Gently rub it on and lick it off!

BODY TREATMENTS
FOR EXFOLIATION

Crushed Cabernet Scrub

The great thing about this scrub is that you can customize it to your liking. Adding more sugar means more buffing power; adding more grape seeds (which give it its name) means more scrubbing power. It smells wonderful as is, or you can add a few drops of your favorite essential oil for its therapeutic properties and luscious scent. Try lemon, geranium, rose, lavender, rosemary, or sandalwood.

¼ cup organic brown sugar
2 tablespoons grape seeds (You can buy grape seeds online, unless you're friendly with a local vineyard!)
At least ⅓ cup grape-seed oil (add more if needed)
¼ cup raw organic honey
A few drops of essential oil (optional)

- Place the sugar and grape seeds in a microwavable bowl.
- Pour on grape-seed oil until the sugar and seeds are fully saturated, then add the honey and essential oil, if using, and mix well.
- Warm the mixture in the microwave for 20 to 30 seconds. (This step is optional.)
- Massage into your skin before stepping into the shower, focusing on areas like the elbows, knees, and the backs of your thighs, and then rinse it off.
- Apply a nourishing body cream when your skin is still damp.

FOR DETOX AND SOOTHING
Detox Bath Salts

This will help remove toxins from your body, too.

8 ounces white vinegar

1 tablespoon baking soda

2 handfuls coarse salt

- Add all ingredients to running bath water.
- Soak for at least 20 minutes.

FOR NAILS
Healthy Nails Potion

This potion will nourish and repair your nails.

1 tablespoon argan oil

1 tablespoon grape-seed oil

1 tablespoon lemon juice

1 to 2 drops lemon essential oil

1 to 2 drops geranium essential oil

1 tablespoon honey

- Mix all ingredients together.
- Apply to nails as needed, and rub it in well.

Glowing Nails Potion

2 tablespoons baking soda
1 ounce lukewarm water

- Mix the baking soda in the water until it's fully dissolved.
- Dip your nails in the mixture for 10 minutes.
- Rinse with water.

FOR HAIR

These easy and inexpensive treatments will leave your hair glorious in no time at all. Try to use one of these masks once a week.

FOR SHINY HAIR

This amazing recipe was handed down to me from my grandmother. It's not the most elegant mixture in the world, but it is very effective. It will leave your hair incredibly nourished, super-shiny, silky, and with loads of body.

Egg Yolk and Rum Mask

2 beaten egg yolks
5 tablespoons dark or light rum
¼ cup olive oil
¼ cup grape-seed oil

- Mix all ingredients until smooth and creamy.
- Apply it to your hair and leave on for at least 30 minutes and up to an hour.
- Shampoo as usual.

Avocado and Olive Oil Mask

2 avocados
A few tablespoons olive oil

- Pulse the avocados and oil in a blender until it turns into a spread.
- Apply to hair and leave on for 10 to 15 minutes.
- Shampoo as usual.

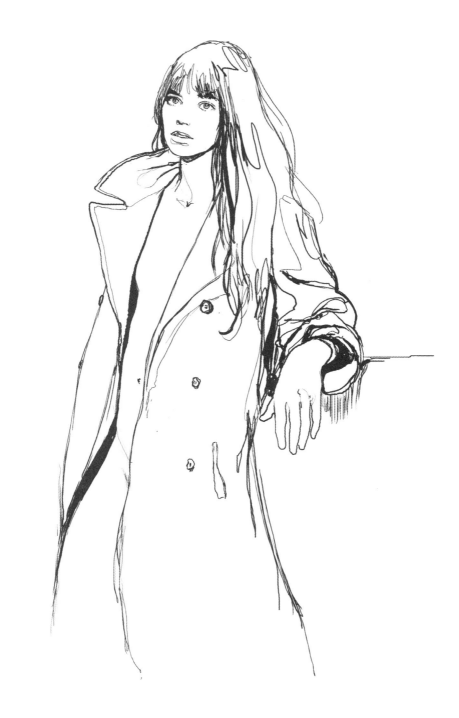

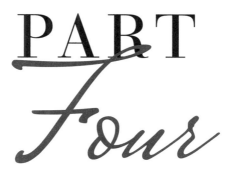

PART
Four

Makeup and Hair
the French Way

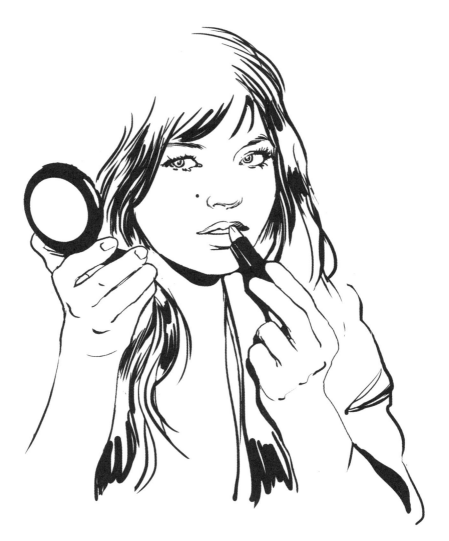

Nine

DO YOUR MAKEUP LIKE THE FRENCH

Going to River Way Ranch Camp in California when I was a teenager was quite the eye-opener. Not only did my friends Nathalie and Tania and I shock our fellow campers, as you know already, when we brazenly sunbathed topless, but we were rendered speechless by a very particular American custom. The *makeup* custom!

Like all my friends and classmates back in Grenoble, we had saved and saved our francs until that magical day when we could saunter into the local *parfumerie* to purchase our very first makeup item: Guerlain's Terracotta blush. It came in a sheer brown compact, and we felt oh-so-grown-up after we ran home and eagerly put it on. Never mind that we didn't exactly have a deft touch, so we did look a little bit *obvious*. No matter—we were young ladies, on the road to blushing womanhood.

So Nathalie, Tania, and I were absolutely flabbergasted when we quickly unpacked our petite French suitcases and then our American bunkmates opened their enormous trunks. There, nestled under their sweaters and pajamas was more makeup than we'd ever seen before. Bags and bags of makeup of all hues and sizes, and cans and cans of hairspray. I still remember how one girl pulled out fourteen of those cans and then carefully lined them up on the shelf over her bed. She could do things with hair I'd never imagined before—I wouldn't be surprised if she grew up to become a hairstylist.

That was the summer I learned how to apply makeup. I had never put so much makeup on in my life and I don't think I have since. Our bunkmates felt terribly sorry for us as we showed them our one little jar of moisturizer and our precious Terracotta bronzer; they couldn't believe that was all we used. They spent endless hours sitting on their beds, playing around with colors, and happily told us about all the time they spent cutting classes so they could do their faces in the bathrooms of their schools, and then quickly wiping everything off before they went back home so they wouldn't get in trouble with their strict parents. They would meticulously do our faces, and we would borrow their eye shadow, and they loved teaching us all their tricks.

Then my friends and I went back to France, and we forgot about all the makeup—because no one we knew ever wore anything more than the usual bronzer and perhaps a swipe of mascara and a hint of lip gloss.

I still barely wore any makeup when I went to university in Paris when I was eighteen. I started to use it in earnest only when I was twenty-three, because Bertrand and I were trying to procure the financing for Caudalie, and I wanted to look older than I was. I borrowed one of my mother's suits and I pulled my hair into a bun and I put on my face so the bankers would see me as a responsible adult—one with a healthy glow. I guess you could say it worked.

This guide, which I've compiled along with suggestions from

the acclaimed French makeup artist Delphine Sicard, should make it easier for you to wear makeup that looks nice but natural.

THE ESSENCE OF FRENCH MAKEUP
START WITH HEALTHY SKIN

No makeup can hide a complexion that isn't fresh and glowing. Always keep your skin hydrated.

Go for the No-Makeup Makeup Look

One thing Frenchwomen admire in American women is how sophisticated their approach to makeup is. You are always on top of all the latest trends in colors and textures and know all the tips to applying the newest products and achieving the trendiest looks. The problem with this approach is that it's so much work and upkeep, and Frenchwomen are simply too lazy to bother.

Frenchwomen just don't go for that much makeup. We haven't ever since the French Revolution, when the royalty who had once loved their white-painted faces and vermillion blush (made from crushed beetles—how *chic!*) and artfully applied black beauty marks scrubbed their faces clean and went into hiding for fear of the guillotine.

That's why the French strive for that done-but-not-done look. You'll wear a bit of makeup but you don't want it to be too noticeable, so we rarely if ever wear any eye shadow other than a barely there neutral or a sweep of subtle eyeliner.

This style of French makeup is very simple, very *chic,* and very easy on the pocketbook. *Oui,* less is more! Even better, it takes only a very little bit of time to master this look—and once you do, your makeup will never let you down, no matter where you're going or what kind of clothing you're wearing.

Streamline Your Routine

Frenchwomen love to streamline their makeup routine, so they spend the least amount of time applying it and the most amount of time looking polished and professional without calling attention to what we've put on our faces. My makeup routine is so simple, as you'll see on page 216, it takes just a minute or two. *Voilà!* I'm done.

Good Grooming Is a Must

This is one area of makeup where I think American women do it better than the French. You have a knack for pulling it all together—your face, your impeccable nails, your beautifully styled hair. A Frenchwoman always cares about looking presentable before she steps out the door, but we have a much higher tolerance for, well, a bit of *messy*. And we justify it by giving one of those infamous Gallic shrugs and claiming that we have so many other things to do (even if that's not quite true).

Play Up Your Best Asset—But Only One at a Time

What do you want to emphasize? Your eyes? Great. Go for smoky eyes with lots of mascara but keep your lips a subtle neutral. Or, if you want to wear a bold red lipstick, apply it carefully, and just wear a light swipe of mascara on your eyes. In other words, only call attention to one asset at a time. And always wear a little bit of a rosy blush on your cheekbones, like NARS Orgasm.

Foundation Is Not the Foundation

Many American women don't feel they've done their makeup unless they wear foundation. Many Frenchwomen wouldn't dream of wearing it. This is one of the biggest differences in our attitude toward makeup.

Creamy foundation was created by Max Factor (yes, he was a real person, and he also coined the word *makeup*) for the movie industry in 1930s Hollywood—the hot lights and the color film stock highlighted every blemish on a performer's face, and his brilliant pancake makeup smoothed out these faces and evened their skin tones so they looked their best. At-home versions of this thick makeup took off like crazy, and American women have been loving their foundation ever since. A good foundation should still, like Max Factor's pancake, even out your skin tone so that any imperfections are less noticeable and key features of your face are more noticeable. But even a good foundation won't enhance your looks if you use too much of it, or if it's visibly "fake." It can, in fact, instantly age you—which is why I wore it to my banker's appointments when I was twenty-three.

No matter what your age, if your skin is in top condition, foundation shouldn't be necessary, especially as it can call attention to pores and wrinkles. We prefer liquid bronzer or tinted moisturizers, which give lighter coverage and a natural glow. A tinted moisturizer contains 15 percent mineral pigments; a foundation 30 percent; and a concealer 40 percent.

The iconic French beauties I wrote about in chapter 1 often wear a lot of foundation when they're walking the red carpet to promote their work—but I've yet to meet any of them who wear foundation when they're out of the public eye. They know they don't need it.

Still, if you like foundation and feel it improves your appearance, go ahead and wear it. There are countless formulations available, so take your time experimenting until you find one that enhances your complexion—without masking it—and go for the sheerest type that still provides the coverage you're looking for.

And don't forget your neck! Foundation should never stop at

your jawline. Moisturize your neck well and then apply foundation from your forehead down to all of your neck area.

Delphine's tip is to choose a foundation with this simple test at the cosmetics counter: Apply a dab on your T-zone and blend it well. Ask for a mirror and go outside to see how well the foundation matches or doesn't match your skin tone. You need to check it in daylight, as indoor lighting (especially the fluorescent lights in department stores) distorts colors and won't give you an accurate reading.

Concealers Are Great at Concealing

Like foundation, concealers should be used sparingly—but when used effectively, they're fantastic products and a must-have for your makeup bag. I never leave home without mine; I apply it in the morning and refresh it again at night if needed when I'm going out.

Apply your concealer under your eyes or on any blemishes, with your ring finger, and blend well. I like to use YSL's famous Touche Éclat, because it is deliberately overloaded with pearlized pigments that reflect light. Look for one that is moisturizing and as close to your skin tone as possible. Or choose a tinted moisturizer, which can have the same concealing effects.

Be Savvy About Primers

Primers are becoming increasingly popular because they can even out your skin tone and give you a smooth surface, but those with a silicone base can be very dehydrating while paradoxically making your face too shiny. Remember, they aren't moisturizers. Look for one that doesn't list silicone as one of the top three ingredients. Try choosing a moisturizer with a primer-like finish instead.

French Beauty Secret

Makeup should never be applied to bare skin. At the very least, you need to apply either a hydrating sunscreen or a moisturizer to provide the proper base for putting on a product, especially foundation or a concealer. This will provide a necessary barrier between the ingredients in makeup, such as color, silicone, and other chemicals that should stay on the surface of your skin rather than be absorbed.

Consider Using Bronzer Rather Than Blush

My first makeup love was a bronzer powder, as you know, and I still use it regularly, especially in colder months when I need something to counteract the gloom and brighten up my cheeks and my spirits. My favorite tinted moisturizers are Caudalie's Teint Divin or Laura Mercier's Tone on Tone, which both give you a healthy, sun-kissed glow. Then I add a bronzing powder and a blush on my cheeks.

For those with very fair skin, bronzer actually looks more natural, as it has a pink undertone rather than the yellow one common to most foundations, making it easier to blend.

If you don't like bronzer, look for a blush in the peach family. This peachy tint is why NARS Orgasm blush is so universally popular. It works on all skin tones.

Take Care of Your Eyelashes

I love seeing women with long, luxurious lashes, but I've yet to meet a Frenchwoman who liked to use false eyelashes or the kind

French Beauty Secret

Left your blush at home and feeling like you need a hint of color? Apply a moisturizer to your cheeks so they're smooth, dab a bit of lipstick on your cheeks, and blend it very well with your fingertips. A little goes a long way—and it's also hard to remove quickly if you use too much, so be very sparing.

of lash extensions or dyes that are done in a salon (and can be dangerous if any of the chemicals get in your eyes). If our lashes are sparse, the French have no qualms about taking supplements that enhance hair growth, like biotin, or using a wonderful conditioning gel called Talika Eyelash Lipocils. My mother used it all the time and she still uses it—and I use it, too, because it really does make your lashes thicker. You can also use an eyelash primer before applying mascara, as this coats your lashes and allows the mascara to intensify.

One bad habit we do have is to overuse eyelash curlers. They're great devices when used properly, but they can cause lash breakage or loss if you push down too hard—so be careful! Go very easy on the pressure and you should be fine.

As for mascara, we prefer a light touch, with mascara used only at the base of your lashes so they look thicker but not fake.

Eye Shadow Is Rarely on Our Makeup List

Frenchwomen rarely use eye shadow, and when we do, we avoid bright colors and stick with soft neutrals instead.

If you like to use eye shadow, stick to subtle neutrals that don't crease; powder formulas tend to crease less than cream formulas.

We do love to use eyeliner; usually a thin line for daytime and a thicker line for a more dramatic nighttime look. I like subtle brown during the day and dramatic black at night.

Don't Forget Your Eyebrows

Eyebrows frame your face, and grooming them is so easy—yet we often neglect them. A polished, shapely brow is actually a huge asset, as it makes you look like you're "done" even if you're just wearing a bit of lipstick, too.

First, take a few seconds to brush your brows. Use an old, cleaned-off mascara brush (or get a new one at a drugstore or beauty supply store) and simply brush them into shape every morning. Then use an eyebrow pencil that matches the shade of your brows. Apply a little bit in short strokes over your brows and you're good to go. If your brows are very sparse or short, fill them in to align with the corners of your eyes.

Waxing is more efficient than tweezing, and if you find some-one who's good at it, stick with her, as overzealous tweezing can make it difficult for the hairs to grow back properly. Threading is also popular and effective, especially in New York, although it's not done in France. Once your brows are well shaped, it's easy to tweeze out the strays. Be conservative when getting your brows done, as if they're too thin, it's very aging, and you don't want to have to faux-pencil them in like Marlene Dietrich had to!

Lips Are for Kissing, Not for Painting

You learned how to take wonderful care of your lips in chapter 6, which is great, because applying lipstick to chapped lips is not something you want to do.

As for lip color, the French are not the great experimenters that American women love to be. We usually stick with a classic red, or a rose-pink or peach that is soft and neutral. Lip color will be bright only if our eyes are not. And we're great fans of lip gloss and shiny formulations as long as the color isn't too bright.

Always Remove Your Makeup at Night

You already know that you're never too tired to take off your makeup at night—but it's worth repeating here. Use a hypoallergenic, oil-based remover, especially if you like waterproof mascara—as long as there is *no* mineral oil in it!—and rinse it off with water. Do this before you wash your face.

MY MAKEUP ROUTINE

As with skincare, my makeup routine is extremely simple. If it takes even five minutes, I'd be surprised.

> **Tinted moisturizer**. I find that using a moisturizer with a hint of color is the ideal replacement for foundation. It gives me coverage without being noticeable, though I do occasionally use foundation if I have a photo shoot that day since it's better at providing coverage in harsh lighting.
>
> **Eyes**. I use Bobbi Brown dark eyeliner followed by Lancôme Hypnose mascara. That's it. For dark circles, I use a YSL concealer, which is opaque enough to hide them without getting cakey. I then add a touch of illuminating white pigments on the inside corners of my eyes as a subtle brightener.

Cheeks. NARS Orgasm is an ideal color for just about anyone's skin tone, as it is a neutral peachy-pink blush that is subtle and real-looking. And of course, who else but a Frenchman would come up with such a sexy name for a blush?

Bronzer. I loved my bronzer as a teenager and I still do. I always use a mineral bronzer. Use a round brush and apply it lightly around the circumference of your face, as if you're outlining a circle. That's the trick that gives you the glow.

Powder. If I need to mattify my T-zone, which doesn't happen often, I use a little bit of Trish McEvoy white finishing powder. Or a natural paper blotter made by Tatcha.

Lipstick. I like NARS Baroque Velvet Gloss lip pencil, which is a soft and subtle Bordeaux red, with a sheer lip gloss on top.

Voilà! Quick, *chic,* and simple.

French Beauty Secret

When I'm on an airplane and ready to sleep, I slide on my eye mask so that it bends my eyelashes upward. It works like an eyelash curler, and when I wake up, my eyes look more open. But you don't have to get on a plane for this trick to work.

DELPHINE'S FRENCH MAKEUP TIPS

In addition to my own secrets, these are Delphine's favorite tips that will help you create a flawless French face:

Q: Is there any kind of makeup that is tricky to use?

> **A:** BB creams—the BB stands for beauty balm or blemish balm—are multitasking products that are very popular, but they can be tricky, as they are designed to give full coverage, making them look obvious, as if you have too much on your skin. It also can be hard to match them to your skin tone. I would recommend a tinted moisturizer instead.

Q: What are your best tips to encourage experimentation? Or should it not be encouraged once you know your best look?

> **A:** It's always interesting to discover and try new products adapted to your skin. Try testing them if there are samples available in a store like Sephora or in a drugstore before you buy them to help figure out what's right for you; or if there are no samples, try them at home and be sure to check in natural light so you get a good idea of how the colors actually look. However, I advise against testing just before an important event! A girl's night, on the other hand, is a great way to get opinions from your friends.

Q: What tools are essential?

> **A:** At least three or four brushes of different sizes/purposes—an eye shadow brush, an eyeliner brush, and one or two blush and foundation brushes—are essential. It's better to

get those of top quality and real hair rather than synthetics, as they will last for years. A powder puff to mattify your skin can be very useful as well, but be sure to clean it frequently.

Q: How do you clean your brushes?

A: Gently wash them with a soft, triple-milled soap, press carefully with a clean towel to remove excess moisture, and dry them lying on a towel on a flat surface. If you stand them up to dry, the water can seep into the handles and eventually warp them.

Q: If you are running late, what should you do?

A: Be sure to hydrate your face, use a bit of concealer on any dark circles or redness, and mascara at the base of your lashes. If you feel confident using a BB cream, that will give you a flawless finish. And be sure to take your red lipstick with you for any touchups and to use as a blush in a pinch.

Q: Would a Frenchwoman ever leave the house without doing her face?

A: No Parisienne I know or that I've worked with would go out without *any* makeup. But they do give their skin a break on the weekends, when they only use a hydrating day cream with a high SPF.

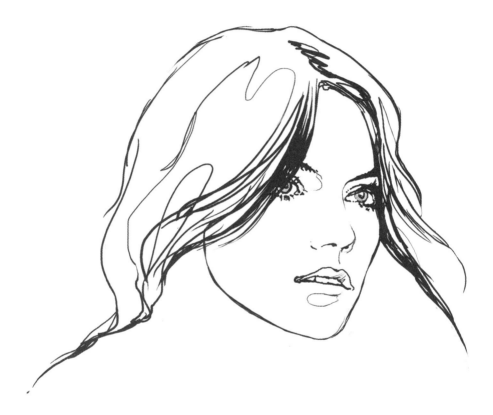

Ten

DO YOUR HAIR LIKE THE FRENCH

Do you know where the term *powder room* comes from? Not from a room where ladies retired after dinner to powder their noses—but where aristocrats of the early seventeenth century went to powder their wigs. They'd sit down, carefully arrange a dressing gown, place a cone of protective paper over their faces, and hope for the best.

Funnily enough, these powder rooms were initially men-only, as Frenchwomen didn't wear those towering and elaborate wigs so beloved of Marie Antoinette until the 1770s. Still, hairstyling was an incredibly important aspect of the life of the French courtiers, and good wigmakers were assured of steady employment—at one point King Louis XIV had forty wigmakers just to tend to his vast collection.

While *coiffeurs* have continued to be an important part of French style and beauty, I wish I could say that their talents extended to me . . . because I'm pretty hopeless about hair! And I think that while Frenchwomen seem to have a knack for finding a style that suits every aspect of their personalities, American women are vastly more interested in and talented about haircare than the French will ever be. On this topic, we need to take the lead from you, although this section will share the many aspects of haircare that we manage to do well, with my tips as well as those of acclaimed French hairstylist Delphine Courteille, who is a regular fixture at the fashion shows for Chanel, Hermès, and Jean Paul Gaultier, and one of the most talented hairdressers of her generation.

THE ESSENCE OF FRENCH HAIRCARE AND STYLING
WHEN IN DOUBT, GO *AU NATUREL*

Frenchwomen are willing to put up the good beauty fight for many things—glowing, healthy skin and a certain radiance being at the top of the list—but one arena where we can be willing to walk away is with our hair. For us, the epitome of hair *chic* is accepting what we've got and making the most of it. We would rather resign ourselves to thick curls than sit for hours being tortured with a toxic hair-straightening treatment; our shelves are not laden with products for this and that and something else. Instead, we get a fantastic cut that enhances whatever kind of hair we have, and we do the minimum possible to keep it in the best shape. We know that the less we do, the better it'll look. And if I'm ever having a bad day, my husband cheers me right up when he says, "Oh, come on, you know I think you look better with your hair naturally curly."

PUT THE BLOW-DRYER AWAY

The easiest way to enhance the *au naturel* look is to go to bed with hair wet from your shower. Use a tiny bit of shampoo, a good conditioner, and say good night; you'll wake up with hair that's got just the texture you want. This also works well when you're at the beach—put your hair in loose braids and the salt water will give your hair extra body and waves as it dries.

More than anything else, this is the number one French beauty secret for hair. The do-nothing hairdo *sans* blow-dryer!

And if that doesn't convince you . . . one of the biggest problems with haircare is the overuse of heat and processing. Every time you blow-dry or flat-iron (and bleach and color) your hair, you're damaging it. Worse, if you spend a lot of time tugging at wet hair when you're styling it, you're at risk for traction alopecia, which is hair loss due to external factors. Do your best to minimize the amount of heat applied to your hair.

MERCI FOR MESSY

The French also have that certain look with their hair—it's deliberately low-maintenance and messy. The great thing about this is that it makes hairstyling a breeze, and you already know how much we love to streamline our beauty routines.

WHEN IN DOUBT, DO A BUN

Frenchwomen tend not to be anywhere near as adventurous with hairstyles as American women are. If anything, they stick to the tried-and-true style of hair long enough to put in a bun. Walk into practically any office in Paris (including Caudalie's) and you will see rows upon rows of perfectly messy buns. When I moved to New York City and went to a meeting with my hair in a bun—and saw all the other women with their beautifully styled hair—I felt very self-conscious. I quickly learned that a stylish outfit and glowing skin will distract from the fact that I'm not brilliant at styling my hair.

YOU DON'T NEED TO WASH YOUR HAIR EVERY DAY

But you do need to wash it—and on this charge, the French are often quite guilty. I clearly remember my mother admonishing me on many occasions about washing my hair every day or even every other day. I have an American friend who studied at the Sorbonne, and she told me how she never forgot her young French instructor, who came to class every Monday with clean and shiny hair—but by the end of the week, Madame's greasy locks were in an appalling state and the dandruff flakes were flying. Clearly, Madame had a once-a-week shampoo habit, and it certainly wasn't enough.

None of the Frenchwomen I know have dirty hair even if they don't wash it every day. They like a bit of texture, so they use a good volumizer or dry shampoo. We know that unless your hair is very oily, you rarely have to wash it every day—and you don't *want* to wash it every day. Or even every other day. Every time you use a detergent-based shampoo (especially one that has sulfates as the top ingredients), your hair will get clean but it will also get dried-out and damaged. All you have to do is rinse it with water between shampoos. Or, if you use shampoo, apply a tiny bit only on your scalp where it's needed. Hair products tend to be concentrated, so you really don't need to use more than a dab the size of a quarter. And contrary to the instructions on a bottle of shampoo, you never have to lather, rinse, and repeat—even if your hair is oily. Squeaky-clean hair is hair that has lost its luster.

CONDITIONING IS MORE IMPORTANT THAN SHAMPOOING

The purpose of conditioner is to improve the luster of your hair by adding much-needed moisture to it and sealing the cuticles. Look for conditioners that won't strip oils from your scalp and that will protect it. Avoid any conditioner with sulfates, and also avoid any conditioner with silicones (such as dimethicone or cyclomethicone)

French Beauty Secret

We love dry shampoo, which of course is better than doing nothing to dirty hair. An effective dry shampoo will keep your hair looking presentable for several days. It also makes your hair easy to style. My favorite brand is Klorane.

as one of the top three ingredients. Your hair should feel soft and manageable afterward, not weighed-down or greasy (if so, you used too much conditioner or the wrong type for your hair.)

The recipes on pages 203 to 204 will help transform your tresses.

DON'T FORGET YOUR SCALP

Do you treat the skin on your scalp with the same lavish attention with which you treat the skin on your face and neck? You should. Regular use of hair masks are a wonderful way to soothe irritated scalps, and the French are also much more likely to use products for scalp health.

Particularly helpful is a product that my mother introduced me to: Phyto's Phytopolléine Universal Elixir Scalp Stimulant. It's primarily composed of essential oils such as rosemary, cyprus, and lemon. It smells incredible and it's great for dry or irritated scalps, and it also stimulates your roots for better hair growth. Apply a dropper full and massage it in well so it soaks in. Leave it on for about twenty minutes and then shampoo as usual. It's one of my favorite hair products.

French Beauty Secret

One of my secret weapons is to apply oil to my hair twenty minutes before shampooing—not just for scalp health but because it does wonders for dry and brittle hair. Oil used therapeutically won't make your hair "oily" or greasy—because you'll wash it out, so don't be afraid to try this. One of my favorites is Caudalie Divine Oil with argan, shea butter, hibiscus, sesame, and polyphenols, but you can use any hair oil you like, especially pure argan oil or unrefined coconut oil.

HAIR COLOR IS FOR COVERING GRAY

Like their American counterparts, French teenagers experiment with color and go from blond to red and back again dozens of times . . . until they don't. While American women fearlessly change color on a regular basis and have a lot of fun doing so, young Frenchwomen stop and listen to their much-more-conservative *mamans* and stick to their natural color. They may get some artful highlights, to be sure, but not much more.

CONSIDER A SUPPLEMENT FOR HAIR GROWTH

My mother has thick hair—and is a bit obsessed with keeping it that way. She knows that the polyphenols in resveratrol are great for stimulating hair growth, and she also takes a supplement every day. The one she likes best is Inneov Masse Capillaire, which contains taurine, zinc, catechins, and green tea polyphenols; brands like Oenobiol or Phyto are good, too. Many Frenchwomen swear by Innéov—but just be warned that this stimulates not only the hair on your head, but the hair everywhere else on your body!

GO TO FRANCE FOR A HAIRCUT

Not long after I moved to New York, I asked a friend who'd lived here for a long time to recommend a great hairdresser. She gave me a few names, and when I called to make an appointment, I nearly dropped the phone each time when I heard the price. Some of them charged close to a thousand dollars—just for a cut! I could practically fly to Paris and back for that price and get a fabulous haircut while I was there, too.

I doubt that haircut prices are as high in other American cities, but hair salons are a terrific bargain in France. There is also an endless supply of wonderful Parisian stylists who will come to your home for no more than about thirty to fifty dollars to cut, blow out, and style your hair.

HOW TO CHOOSE A GOOD HAIR BRAND

Frenchwomen, who are very loyal to their hairdressers, often ask them for advice about choosing the products best suited to their hair. American women often do the same, but as there are so many incredible brands in America, choosing the right one can be daunting.

The easiest way to narrow your choices is to avoid any shampoo with sulfates. They're the most common ingredient in many shampoos, either as sodium laurel or sodium laureth sulfate. That's because they are effective detergents that instantly lather up a lot—and Americans love their bubbles. But sulfates are also the kind of detergents with which you wash your dishes or your car. They might foam up on command but they are harsh and drying.

Silicone is another ingredient that suits some women but not others. It coats your hair and makes it shiny and slippery, but it's not an effective conditioner. It's best used for thick or coarse hair, as it can instantly weigh down fine hair, making it look limp and even greasy.

My recommendation is to use any of the French brands, such as Phyto, René Furturer, Leonor Greyl, and Christophe Robin, which have a wide range of items for very specific needs.

HOW I TAKE CARE OF MY HAIR

My hair is a challenge, especially in the summer, when I love water sports even while knowing that chlorine and sun exposure can leave your hair fried, dry, and frizzy. It needs nourishing and moisture.

Washing

Use a shampoo you like that is free of sulfates, as they dehydrate your hair and scalp. You need only a dime-size amount. American women tend to use way too much shampoo and overclean their hair, which leaves it primed for dryness and flyaways.

Conditioning

Use a lightweight conditioner and leave it on while you wash your body. If I'm on the road and don't have time to whip up one of the hair masks on pages 203 to 204, I like to use René Furterer Karité shea butter mask or Ojon's oil preshampoo.

Haircare and Styling Products

As you know, I am a hairstyling minimalist. Mostly all I do is apply pure organic argan oil and a blend of grape-seed oil, hibiscus oil, and liquid shea butter to moisturize the ends—and then I put it in a bun!

French Beauty Secret

Probably the most shared secret among my friends—in other words, something all French-women know—is how to get shiny hair. Simply rinse it with vinegar after shampooing. The smell doesn't linger and it costs pennies. And if you're a blond, you can finish that off with a rinse made of chamomile tea, which tones down brassiness (it's especially good after a swim in a chlorinated pool). Then use the leftover tea bags as a puffiness remover for your eyes. Place the wet tea bags on your eyes, lie down for a few minutes, and you'll look a lot more refreshed.

DELPHINE'S FRENCH HAIRSTYLING TIPS

Q: What is the most important/iconic aspect of French hairstyling?

A: For Frenchwomen, what really matters is style—fashion style and haircut style. We go for a look that is simple and natural without looking "done."

Q: Are Frenchwomen adventurous with their hair, or do they stick to pretty much the same thing?

A: Frenchwomen who love fashion will follow the trends, such as beach waves or a short bob. These are risks but always with the "French touch"—in which everything is calculated but the style still looks natural. Frenchwomen don't like it if people notice they came from the hairdresser—it's the equivalent of the no-makeup makeup look for hair.

Q: How do styles evolve as women grow older?

A: Even older Frenchwomen want to stay natural. They like it when their haircut lasts for a long time. If they have dark hair, they will want to lighten their hair for less maintenance, as it's easier to hide the gray that way. They want to look youthful but also age-appropriate.

Q: Do the French color their hair as much as Americans do?

A: Frenchwomen color their hair as much as American women. But French colorists will use more natural products adapted to the demand: no jet-black, no fake chestnut, no burgundy red, no ombré. Just natural-looking highlights that make hair look as if it's been sun-kissed. Women often bring in pictures of themselves when they were younger and ask for the same color—they know it will suit their skin tone.

Q: What does a Frenchwoman do when she sees that first gray hair?

A: Most of them hide it!

Q: Is there a special kind of hairstyling product that Frenchwomen love or don't use?

A: We love good conditioners, and especially go for texturizing products, such as a volumizing powder or sea salt spray. One product we never use is hair gel.

Q: What kind of brushes are the best?

A: I like Y. S. Park flat brushes made in Japan, or Mason Pearson brushes, which are sold in local *pharmacies*.

Q: Is there anything the French think about what Americans do to their hair that is just astonishing or something they'd never try?

A: Frenchwomen often say, "Please don't do the Dallas brushing to me"—which means, "Please do not give me big hair or a super-volumizing blow-dry." For us, less is more.

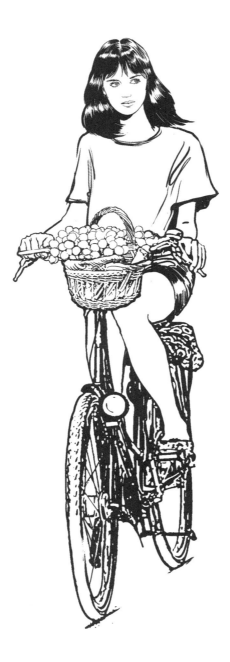

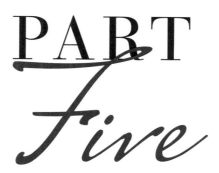

PART Five

The Essentials of the
Three-Day Grape Cleanse

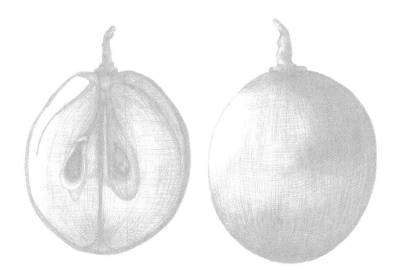

Eleven

THE GRAPE CLEANSE

I first did the Grape Cleanse in 1998, when I was researching and writing my first book, *La Santé par le Raisin* (or *Health from the Grape*), and I discovered the history of the therapeutic use of grapes, and that many of the people who loved this process wrote extensively about it. It's incredibly simple. For several days—or for longer, if you choose—all you eat are grapes. A *lot* of grapes!

Not surprisingly, I was very curious, so I decided to try the cleanse for myself. The day before I started, I ate only fruits and vegetables to get my body ready; I didn't drink coffee at the time so I wasn't worried about caffeine withdrawal. Then I bought enormous bunches of beautifully ripe, organic red and white grapes for variety. (It's easier to find the seeded varieties in France.) I also drank green tea throughout.

Yes, by day three I was a bit bored looking at another grape—I felt the same way whenever I had done a juice cleanse in the past, too—but I felt great all the way. I was totally energized and felt clean and detoxified. My belly became quite flat, but the most interesting thing was the quality of my skin. I'd literally never seen it like that before—with this amazing, soft texture and glow. It had the same glow you see in ads with supermodels and their petal-perfect skin, except I knew I wasn't Photoshopped!

The day after I finished, I ate only fruit and vegetables, but no more grapes. I felt incredible. I hadn't lost much weight, but I still felt *lighter*. So read on, as you might want to try this cleanse for yourself.

THE POWER OF THE GRAPE

The humble little grape is an amazing fruit—one of the most potent in history. It's even nicknamed the vegetal milk because its nutritional composition is so complete.

Found in their wild state in many parts of the world, the vines that produce grapes for eating and wine have been domesticated for centuries. Can you imagine reading the Bible, or studying the ancient Greeks and Romans without the copious references to wine? In sixteenth-century France, King Louis XIV demanded the finest wines at his vast table, and he had his favorite grapes packed carefully in straw before being shipped to his court in crates borne by mules and horses. It wasn't until the nineteenth century, though, that grapes became a regularly eaten fruit—and now, it's hard to imagine a world or a kitchen without them.

THE COMPOSITION AND NUTRITIONAL VALUE OF GRAPES

Each bunch of grapes has two distinct sections: the stem and the actual fruit, or the berry of the grape. The berry consists of the skin, a juicy pulp, and a cluster of seeds. It is covered by a powder formed by small waxy flakes that the grape produces in order to protect itself from rain and the elements. A freshly picked grape will be covered in this powder, and it's easily removed with the tip of your finger. If you see it on your grapes, that's a good thing—it shows that the fruit hasn't been processed and is at the peak of its freshness. Another way to check for freshness is a stem that is extremely green and firm.

The delectable grape aroma comes from the skin itself. Different grapes have different aromas, depending on the soil, climate, and how the grapes are grown.

Along with figs, grapes are one of the most calorie-dense and sugar-laden fruits, containing approximately 64 to 72 calories per 3.5 ounces. Because grapes are laden with easily assimilated fruit sugars, they are ideal for anyone who needs a burst of energy.

Each 100 grams (a little over ¾ cup) of grapes contains the following:

Water: 78 to 82 grams

Carbohydrates (mainly glucose and fructose): 16 to 18 grams

Protein: 0.7 gram

Malic acid: 0.5 to 2 grams

Iron: 0.5 gram

Tartaric acid: 0.3 to 0.7 gram

Fatty substances: 0.3 gram

Potassium: 183 milligrams

Calcium: 15 milligrams

Citric acid: 20 to 50 milligrams

Phosphorus: 20 milligrams

Magnesium: 9 milligrams

Sulfur: 8 milligrams

Sodium: 3 milligrams

Vitamin C: 0.5 to 11 milligrams

Niacin: 0.3 milligram

Copper: 0.1 milligram

Vitamin A: 0.05 milligram

Vitamin B_1 (thiamine): 0.05 milligram

Vitamin B_2 (riboflavin): 0.03 milligram

Vitamin B_5: 0.05 milligram

Their mineral content, drawn from the soil, is potent, making them a good source of mineral salts, which help alkalinize the blood (many of us are too acidic, which alters the body's natural pH balance, often due to eating a lot of meat), and organic acids, which bring a refreshing tartness to the otherwise sweet berry. Grape-seed oil is particularly nutritious, high in polyunsaturated fats and vitamin E.

What makes grapes so effective in cures and detoxes is their tremendous ability to act as purifier and diuretic. Due to high levels of water, potassium, and fiber, grapes help stimulate the entire digestive system, helping your body eliminate waste and cleanse its organs. And where grapes shine the most, of course, is with their polyphenol content, found in the skins, stems, and especially the seeds, that remove the free radicals that can cause so much damage inside your cells, leading to premature aging.

ORIGINS OF THE GRAPE CURE

Although the potent goodness of the grape has been known about since antiquity, in the writings of the Romans Pliny and Galien, it wasn't until the eighteenth century that doctors started recommending a grape cure—which is a longer process than the short three-day cleanse I do every year—to their patients. The pioneer for using grapes as a cure was a French professor of medicine named Desbois de Rochefort. "After much feedback from practitioners including myself, it has been proven that grapes are the best detoxifiers for the spleen," he wrote in 1789. "It is very good for the obstruction of abdominal viscus, the rebellious yellowing, the quartan fever with the obstruction of the lower stomach, especially in the black diseases, hypochondria, and other cutaneous diseases, as it is an excellent purifier."

It still took another 150 years before the medical establishment recognized these properties, however. At that point, when medical journals began to discuss the therapeutic values of grapes, the upper classes of Europe started flocking to local spas for thermal cures and grape detoxes. By the end of the nineteenth century, these detoxes were extremely popular in Germany, Switzerland, Poland, Russia, and Italy, with luxe hotels in locations like Dürkheim in Bavaria and the Veytaux near Lake Geneva.

The French needed a bit of time to catch up, and this took place in the town of Moissac, known for its thermal springs and golden grapes. The first French spa (*soins thérapeutique*) to offer grape detoxes as well as servings of delicious grape juice in a small clubhouse—called an *uvarium*—was established on the banks of the Tarn River in 1927. These cures were primarily targeted to those who were overweight or obese, as well as for gout, constipation, skin disorders, and liver and kidney diseases. Spa guests were instructed to eat up to five pounds of grapes every day or to drink grape juice, and the cure usually lasted at least a month, depending on the medical needs.

The grape cure became so popular that other spas quickly sprung up, such as Fort de L'eau and Philippeville in Algeria, Baden-Baden in Germany, Avignon and Colmar in France, Merano and Rome in Italy, as well in as many Romanian cities. A French federation for the grape cure–oriented spas was even formed in France, but World War II interrupted plans for expansion. After the war, with the advent of modern medicine and more "scientific" treatments, most people lost interest in natural, holistic therapies and thermal cures. Grape detoxes became less and less popular and are now offered at only a few locations; there are spas in the South Tyrol, Moldavia, Bolzano in Italy, and, of course, at the Caudalie spa in Bordeaux at Les Sources de Caudalie.

JOHANNA BRANDT AND THE GRAPE CURE

The grape cure would likely have faded away completely were it not for a South African nurse named Johanna Brandt. Diagnosed with stomach cancer in 1922, she became increasingly ill until her situation was dire three years later. She followed an intensive six-week grape cure—and her cancer disappeared. "The more the body is overrun with toxins, poison, and trash, the more likely it is for a pathology to develop. The detox cleanses the body as well as fights against diseases," she wrote in her book, *The Grape Cure*.

But because Johanna never divulged her cancer treatment and what, precisely, she ate (or didn't eat) on her grape cure, no one will ever know for certain why her cancer was healed. It could have been the grapes, or a fluke, or something else, but Johanna was absolutely convinced it was the grapes. She set sail for America in 1928 to try to convince doctors and the media about her astonishing experience. Finally, a naturopathy publication published her story, and it finally sparked worldwide interest.

Three decades later, another South African, Basil Shackleton, also claimed he had cured his kidney disease with grapes. In his book, *The Grape Cure: A Living Testament*, he explained how antibiotics couldn't help him, so he used grapes and fasting—which is what animals do when they're sick, and is a long-known method for allowing the digestive system to have a break—to heal himself. His theories were shared by other naturopathic healers, and they have fine-tuned Basil's methods ever since, giving hope to many who've been told their illnesses were untreatable.

It must be said, of course, that the Grape Cleanse I love to undergo every year is not a medical treatment, and although we've covered the amazing research into how various properties of grapes, particularly polyphenols, can fight the aging process, there is no scientific evidence that a grape detox can cure cancer or other serious maladies. And, as with skin conditions, self-diagnosis of your health can have lethal results—the mole you thought was nothing could be a melanoma, and the fatigue could mean a thyroid imbalance . . . or they could be completely benign. Before undertaking any kind of cure, fast, cleanse, or radical change in eating habits, consult your physician, especially if you have an underlying medical condition. This is particularly important if you have any blood sugar–related illness such as diabetes.

Use the Grape Cleanse as intended, though, and I hope you will find, as I have, that this short-term detox will make you feel absolutely incredible.

DOES A GRAPE CURE REALLY WORK?

In 1990, the Terre Vivante association (or Living Land, a French organization devoted to agriculture and farming in rural areas) conducted a controlled scientific study on approximately five hundred people and demonstrated that the grape cure is an effective way to revitalize the body, as you'll see in detail in the next section. This cure is a mono-diet, meaning you eat only one food. (Mono-diets can be either a fruit, a vegetable, or a grain.) For at least two centuries, mono-diets have been known as one of the most effective natural therapies for optimal health, as they provide our bodies a break from stresses both external (air, water, noise, nitrates, pesticides) and internal (preservatives, coloring, medications, stimulants and alcohol, and too much acid-forming food that upsets the body's natural balance).

In addition, a mono-diet gives your body a digestive rest between meals; because only one food is eaten, it eases stress on the organs that are used to purify your blood as well as deal with your body's waste—your skin, first and foremost, as well as your gallbladder, liver, kidneys, and intestines.

Although 10 percent of the study's participants thought the cure was frustrating and had no benefits, a resounding 90 percent thought otherwise. They saw a drastic, positive change in their overall energy level and condition, using words like *energetic, extra-strength, dynamic, euphoric,* and *well-being* to describe how they felt after the cure.

In my own experience, I've found that many people are skeptical before they start even a very short Grape Cleanse, because it challenges all the rules of most cleanses you're familiar with. And yet the vast majority of those who'd been exhausted before the cure found themselves completely revitalized. They slept better and continued to sleep better, and they often found their aches and pains, sinus problems, and headaches to be gone as well.

BENEFITS OF THE THREE-DAY GRAPE CLEANSE

I always do the Grape Cleanse for only three days. At the spas and resorts where the grape cure is still used, it often takes place over ten days or more, where guests not only can be medically supervised but also have nothing more stressful to do than concentrate on relaxation. (This usually doesn't happen at the Caudalie Spa in Les Sources de Caudalie Bordeaux, as we have a two-stars-Michelin-awarded chef and so much incredible wine on-site that our guests usually don't want to sacrifice these wonderful meals.) And because they don't often have access to nearby supermarkets or restaurants, and have the full support of the staff and the other guests also doing a mono-diet, it's much easier to stick to a longer grape cure when you are at a spa or away from your regular routine. Those who sign on for a cure rather than a short cleanse usually do so not only for health reasons but also because it will usually lead to weight loss, and that's a powerful incentive.

Needless to say, most working women find it hard to take a day off, much less a few weeks to do a cure, even though it will be wonderful for their health. If you feel great after three days on the Grape Cleanse and want to continue, go ahead and try it—you can stop at any time. (Always check with your physician first, especially if you have any preexisting medical condition or take certain medications.) My sister once did the grape cure for fourteen days; her skin was incredible and she did lose weight, but for me, a three-day cleanse is long enough to reap all the amazing benefits.

That's because the Three-Day Grape Cleanse is an ideal way to not only kick-start your beauty routine but also make you feel a lot better, too. It is far less expensive than other cleanses (some juice cleanses can cost more than eating out at an expensive restaurant); it takes no time at all to prepare, other than buying and washing the grapes; and it is impossible to do "wrong," because all you're eating is fresh grapes. The cleanse might be short, but it can have immediate effects:

- Improvements in your skin. When you eat only grapes for three days, you're giving your digestive system a rest since it doesn't have to work hard to process fats or protein. As a result, toxins that have built up can be eliminated. You might actually notice a few breakouts or itchiness over the first day or two as this is happening, though this has never happened to me. In fact, I noticed that my skin was flawless within twenty-four hours. By day three, you should have brighter and more luminous skin, with no breakouts and an even texture.

- Less fatigue and stress. Most of the people who took part in the controlled Terre Vivante study said they were exhausted and stressed before they started the cure but felt a lot more invigorated afterward. This is because a Grape Cleanse or cure gives not only your digestive system a break, but also your nervous system. You may find yourself with a minor headache the first day as your body adjusts, but I've never had one and feel so much more vital and energized afterward. This is especially true for coffee drinkers, as you are not supposed to drink caffeine on the cure and spontaneous withdrawal can cause headaches and irritability. If you're planning a cure, wean yourself off coffee in advance (we'll discuss this more later in the chapter).

- Insomnia. Because you are giving your body such a well-deserved break during the cleanse, its natural stress levels are going to decline. Plus you won't be ingesting anything that is a stimulant, such as caffeine, refined sugar, or alcohol. This should lead to deeper and more refreshing sleep not only during the three days but afterward as well. I've always fallen right asleep and slept like a baby whenever I do the cleanse.

- Waste elimination. Fiber-rich vegetables, legumes, and fruits get your bowels working properly, so eating nothing but grapes, which have high levels of fiber, for three days should definitely have a gentle laxative effect. You'll also notice that grapes have a diuretic effect, which also helps eliminate waste from your body. Stimulating your body's elimination is part of what makes the Grape Cleanse such a useful detox for your entire body.

- An improved sense of taste and smell. I'm not sure why this happens, but I love anything that enhances my senses. Perhaps my taste buds got some time off like the rest of my body and rewarded me as a result. And that first glass of red wine I drink when I'm back to my regular dinnertime meal is even more delicious.

- Improved eating habits. The Three-Day Grape Cleanse is *not* a weight-loss treatment. Eating only grapes for a few days may well help you lose a few pounds, but this would primarily be water weight, which is quickly gained back when you start eating normally again. If you do the longer grape cure for weeks or even months, then, yes, you will lose weight—but you should do a long cure only under medical supervision.

Apart from how wonderful your skin will look, one of the best rewards of this quick cleanse is how it helps you recognize your eating habits and appreciate what true hunger is. Take a look at your hunger triggers and you'll notice how much you actually *do* eat during the day, and when, and why. Following a restrictive plan like the Grape Cleanse is something nearly everyone can manage for three days and will help you realize that you don't actually *need* that morning bagel or afternoon snack to thrive throughout the day. Once you understand this, you can start to eat like the French!

HOW TO DO THE THREE-DAY GRAPE CLEANSE

Three of my favorite days of the year are the ones I take for the Grape Cleanse. I've been doing this every fall since 1998, except when I've been pregnant.

BEFORE YOU START THE THREE-DAY GRAPE CLEANSE

Congratulations on deciding to do this cleanse! I hope it makes you feel as wonderful as I feel when it's done. As I mentioned above, always clear this detox with your doctor before you start, especially if you have any underlying health issues.

Spending the time necessary to properly prepare for the cleanse will make it even easier and more productive, so follow these tips:

- The best time to do this cleanse is when you are able to take it easy and rest—a vacation or a weekend. Plan it around the three-day period when you will be at home with, hopefully, minimal stress. If you have sudden plans due to changes at work or with your family, push it back to a less fraught time, if possible.

- Ideally, you should do the cleanse when the grapes are harvested, which is in the fall, as they are at their best, full of nutrients, and super-fresh. If the fall isn't convenient, that's fine. Since food is now shipped all over the world and growing seasons are increasingly interchangeable, you can find fresh, nutritious grapes year-round. Still, try your utmost to time your cleanse to the early fall.

- Make sure you can find red grapes that are organic and have seeds, which as you know are the most nutritious part of the grape. If you can't find organic grapes near you, be sure to wash the ones you have bought thoroughly to remove any pesticide residues. You can make a rinse with a few tablespoons of wine vinegar mixed into a quart of water, which will remove impurities and any dirt.

- The grapes should be very ripe but not mushy; unripe grapes are not only sour but also can upset your stomach. Look for varieties that are as deeply colored as possible, as they will have the most nutrients.

- You can choose as many different varieties of grapes as you can find, but remember that the darker the skin, the more polyphenols and other nutrients they contain.

- Swallow the seeds without chewing them, as they can be irritating to the inside of your mouth and your gums if chewed.

- Make sure to buy enough grapes! You are going to be eating a lot of them, and you don't want to run out halfway through. Most people eat anywhere from four to six (or more) *pounds* of grapes each day. That might sound like a lot, but it really isn't considering that's all you'll be ingesting.

- One of the most important steps is to eat as clean a diet as possible for at least a week or more, primarily fruit and vegetables and whole grains. This will get your digestive juices flowing and prime your body for the cleanse. Do your best to avoid red meat, heavy meals, alcohol (even your one glass of red wine at dinner, if you usually have it), coffee or any other caffeinated drinks, and chocolate or any other food with caffeine in it. If you drink a lot of coffee or tea, try to wean yourself off gradually so you don't suffer from caffeine withdrawal. An easy way to do this is to start mixing decaf with your regular coffee, and gradually add more decaf to the mix. Also start drinking more green tea as a replacement.

- Relax! Part of the fun of the Grape Cleanse is seeing it as an adventure—not just for your body, but for your mind and spirit, too. If you've never tried a cleanse or a program like this before, I think you will be amazed at how quickly you can adjust and how quickly your "hunger" will diminish. If you're not in the mood when you thought you would be, or if you're doing it because someone told you to, it's harder to feel good about the process. If so, you might want to push your start date back to a more opportune time. You might also want to have a friend or two do the cleanse with you so you can compare notes and enjoy the process together.

WHAT TO DO DURING THE CLEANSE
DAY ONE

When you start, eat only grapes. Eat the skins *and* the seeds.

- Drink only water, herbal tea, green tea, or Rooibos tea.

- It's better to eat small "meals" of grapes throughout the day rather than sticking to the typical breakfast, lunch, and dinner meals. The ideal schedule is to drink two large glasses of water when you get up, followed by grapes within the next half hour, and then at three-hour intervals during the day. For example, if you at got up at 7:30 A.M., drink your water, then eat your grapes at 8:00 A.M., 11:00 A.M., 2:00 P.M., 5:00 P.M., and 8:00 P.M.

- If you're still hungry between those times, eat more grapes! It's completely okay to nibble if you feel the need. Just don't eat the grapes too quickly, even if you are hungry. Take your time, and savor each little grape, especially the super-nutritious skin. This will help curb any hunger pangs and aid your digestion.

- Expect to eat anywhere from two to more than five pounds of grapes. There is no set figure; it depends on your individual appetite.

- On an empty stomach, at some point during the day, drink eight ounces of freshly squeezed, unsweetened grape juice. I make my own in a blender, as this pulverizes the nutritious skins and seeds.

- Try to keep your regular stress level at a minimum, if at all possible. In other words, don't volunteer for a new project at work. Hopefully, you'll be doing the cleanse over a weekend, so you'll have more time to relax. Really do your utmost to take it easy.

- Go to bed earlier than usual if possible. A soothing hot bath before bed will help you sleep, too.

DAY TWO

The first and second days of any cleanse are always the most difficult, as your body adjusts to being fed a single food and gets rid of the toxins that were there before you started the mono-diet. You might wake up with a headache or a few spots on your skin. You might be tired and maybe even a little grumpy, and you might feel unusually cold. Don't worry—these are signs that the detox is working, and they'll soon go away.

- Follow the same eating and drinking schedule as Day One.

- As you know, black and dark-red grapes have the most nutrients, but if your stomach is acting up, eat seeded green grapes, which are easier to digest.

- Do a little bit of gentle exercise, if at all possible. A long walk is ideal.

DAY THREE

Follow the same eating and drinking schedule as Day One.

- You should be feeling energized and vibrant, and your skin will look amazing.

AFTER THE CLEANSE

When the three days are over, congratulate yourself!

- You will still feel energized, and you will be sleeping better, too.

- After you finish the detox, keep drinking fresh, unsweetened grape juice on an empty stomach, approximately twenty minutes before breakfast, for three days. This will help reinforce the benefits of the cleanse.

- Ease yourself back into regular eating with fresh, unprocessed foods and drinks that are easy to digest. Try dairy products like unsweetened Greek yogurt or cottage cheese, small amounts of whole grains such as oatmeal, and light protein such as fish or chicken. Try to ease yourself back into the coffee habit, too, if you have one. Avoid anything processed and laden with preservatives, chemicals, and/or trans fats; anything fried; or anything made with white sugar and white flour, such as pastries or desserts. (If you're like me, you'll be craving savory, not sweet foods. I love to eat a salad with fresh vinaigrette, some ratatouille, and sushi, which is light and clean yet filling, after my cleanse.)

  In other words, do not go out for a steak or fried-chicken dinner on Day Four, or your body might rebel. You want to give your body time to adjust after a mono-diet, so expect that to happen within half the time of the cleanse's length (which is one and a half to two days).

- If you're like many people who've done the Grape Cleanse, you'll find that your appetite for the food you once thought you couldn't live without has greatly diminished—even after only three days. I think that our bodies are usually under so much assault from the food we eat and the environment we live in that they are so thrilled to have a break, and they send the message to our brains to keep it going as long as possible. This may explain why more than half of the people who were participants in the Terre Vivante study found it easy to change their eating habits. They ate fewer sweets, dairy, meat, and coffee and tea, while eating more unprocessed vegetables, whole grains, fruits, and other raw foods. Equally important is that they ate far less food, too.

- I recommend doing the Grape Cleanse once a year. It's an ideal way to treat your body well, improve your energy and your skin, and take a break from your regular eating habits.

IN CONCLUSION

When I was about fifteen, I decided to go to Paris to visit my friend Tania, who'd moved there several years before. I bought a puffy light-blue skirt, thinking I looked super-fancy and amazing, and took the train, counting the minutes till I arrived. Tania met me on the platform in Gare de Lyon, and her face went from crazy happy to see me to crestfallen as soon as she saw how I looked.

"You cannot *possibly* be seen on the streets with me like *that*," she hurriedly said. "Please tell me you have some cash on you so we can go shopping."

I nodded, and relief flooded her eyes. She put her sweater around my shoulders and quickly walked me to SAP, a boutique in the Sixteenth Arrondissement, where she had me buy a stiff new pair of slightly baggy Levi's 501 jeans, which was what everyone was wearing at the time. Then she pointed me in the direction of the shirts, and put me in a simple white cotton button-down. I wore the outfit out of the store and she stuffed my beautiful blue skirt in the bottom of my handbag.

Then she took a good look at my face, which was completely bare, and took me into the ladies' room of a nearby café, where she pulled out her makeup bag. A swift sweep of Guerlain Terracotta on my face, a soft peachy pink gloss on my lips, and a little mascara on my lashes, *et voilà!* In just a few minutes, she had done a complete makeover. I wasn't insulted—*au contraire!* I was totally impressed with her Parisian fashion and beauty savvy.

I hope you have found this book to be the equivalent of what Tania did for me. She shared her secrets and transformed me in a flash. All these years later, I still have a very simple, quick, and effective beauty routine in the morning so that I look like myself, but just a little bit better and more polished. And I still love to wear simple and *chic* white shirts and denim.

Here's to French beauty!

ACKNOWLEDGMENTS

I would like to thank all of the following:

My better half, a great dad, lover, best friend, and business partner, Bertrand, who pushed me to write this book.

My kids, Paul, Louise, and Marion, who inspire me, even though they may drive me crazy sometimes.

My sister, Alice, who is the coolest.

My wise father, who encouraged me to follow my passion and pushed us to create our company. I hope I inherited his legendary common sense.

My mother, for her drive and her all-time inspirational high energy.

My maternal grandparents: Yvonne, who was the incarnation of kindness, and who made the best wild strawberry jams; and Maurice, for teaching me about plants and nature.

ACKNOWLEDGMENTS

My paternal grandma, "Mam," for being an inspirational entrepreneur and a strong independent woman.

My lifelong friends Tania and Nathalie. We had fun growing up together, and I learned a lot with you.

Professor Joseph Vercauteren, the genius scientist behind Caudalie, who started it all. And Professor David Sinclair of Harvard Medical School, for finding the next Caudalie reverse-aging molecules. You both rock—thanks to you we are going to look younger longer!

Dr. Bernard Hertzog for discovering the secret recipe of the Beauty Elixir of Queen Isabelle of Hungary.

Dr. Heidi Waldorf, Régine Berthelot, Patricia Manissier, Agnès Lefur, Delphine Sicard, and Delphine Courteille for your contributions to this book. I consider you the best pros in your fields.

Thank you to everyone at Caudalie for being such an amazing team: Stéphane Enouf (our visionary general manager), Aude Minc, Emmanuelle Daumesnil, Mathilde Stronher, Aurélie Nattée, Hélène Salat-Baroux, Edouard Nicol, Angélique Mahot, Cécile Ossola, Marine Hery, William Addi, Hervé Sachot, and Odile Grossman.

Thank you Caudalie US for helping me make this book happen: Carole Silverman (our charismatic CEO), Desiree Lestingi, Ellen To, Liz Shoer, Thea Kocher, Emilie Bondu, and Antoine Lefort.

Thank you for sharing your beauty secrets with me : Laure Castets, Aurélie Steinmetz, Alix Ligot, Emily Le Moult, Gaëlle Vassilev, and Delphine Duffours.

Thank you, Karen Moline, for helping me write this book in English. I think you are secretly French.

ACKNOWLEDGMENTS

Thank you to my PR, Alison Brod and her team, and Sharra Lebov and Cara Maiman Hilfer.

Maxime Poiblanc, for your beautiful photo.

My agent, Steve Troha, and his assistant, Dado Derviskadic, at Folio Literary Management.

Everyone at Gotham. Brooke Carey, our tireless Francophile editor; Lucia Watson, thank you so much for your patience. Monica Benalcazar and Spring Hoteling, whom I drove crazy with my sense of detail, and Lindsay Gordon, Caroline Sutton, Megan Newman, Lauren Marino, Casey Maloney, Gabrielle Campo, Pi Pemberton, and Farin Schlussel.

INDEX OF RECIPES BY INGREDIENT

1% FOR THE PLANET | MEMBER

Anyone who purchases *The French Beauty Solution* contributes to protecting the planet, because the author is donating a portion of her proceeds from the sale of this book to "1% for the Planet." As a member of "1% for the Planet" since March 2012, Caudalie donates 1 percent of its global sales to ecological NGOs that work in the most threatening regions of the world. From 2012 to the end of 2015, a total of 440,000 trees will be planted in the Andean Amazon and Brazil in cooperation with NGOs Coeur de Forêt and Nordesta. In addition, 36,000 hectares of natural forest will be protected on the island of Sumatra in Indonesia with WWF. Finally, by the end of 2015, 200,000 trees will be planted in Thailand on the Isaan plateau in cooperation with Alter Eco.